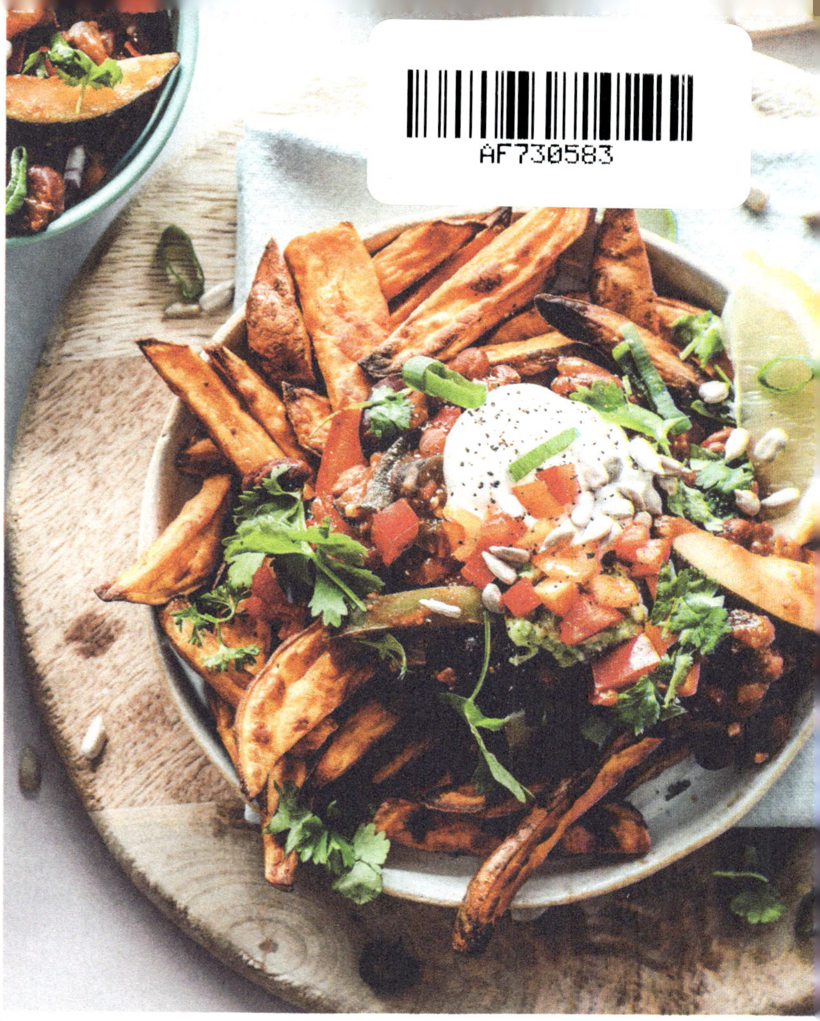

Daily Food & Reflection Diary

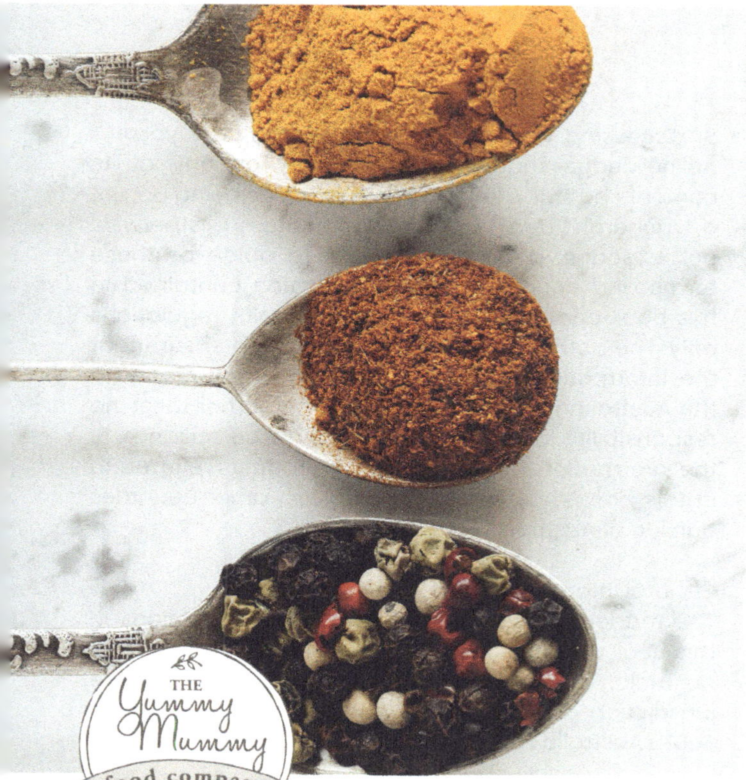

Tracking Your Nutrition for Better Health During Postpartum

THE Yummy Mummy food company

THE MAKE MORE MILK Method

WWW.YUMMYMUMMYFOOD.COM.AU

First edition, 2023
Self-published by The Yummy Mummy Food Company
www.yummymummyfood.com.au

Postpartum Essentials Breastfeeding Nutrition Daily Food & Reflection Journal
ISBN 978-0-6459424-2-2

Yummy Mummy Food Company is proudly Australian made & owned.

Author: Kelly Northey

Disclaimer

General disclaimer
The authors and contributors review all content and have made reasonable efforts to ensure that all information provided is appropriate, accurate, and up-to-date, however make no warranty. The author does not accept any liability to any person for any injury, loss, damage or consequences incurred by use of or in reliance on the information provided in this book. The information in this book is not intended to replace the advice of your healthcare practitioner. It does not take into account your individual health, medical, physical, psychological or emotional situation. The information in this book is designed to provide a basic understanding of the topics discussed. Before acting or using any of the information provided in this book you must have regard to your own personal situation and needs and consider if this information is right for you. This book should not be used to diagnose a suspected medical condition and for a diagnosis you must consult with your health care professional.

By accessing, viewing or purchasing this book you:
Acknowledge that you will not rely on any of its contents but will treat the information as being only of a general and informative nature. Otherwise acknowledge, accept and agree to abide by these terms and conditions. The information contained in this book complies with Australian health regulations only. The author has made every effort to ensure that the information provided in this book comples with the Australian health regulations. The author takes no responsibility for the accuracy or legal compliance of the information in other countries. Products referred to in this book may not be available in other countries outside of Australia.

General Information and Waiver:
The reader agrees that the terms and conditions in this book are governed by the laws of South Australia, Australia. The reader agrees to the exclusive jurisdiction of the Courts located within the state of South Australia for any disputes.

MEET YOUR POSTPARTUM NUTRITION PROFESSIONAL

Meet Kelly Northey Certified Postpartum Nutrition Professional & Founder of the Yummy Mummy Food Company

With a deep passion for empowering mothers through founding the Yummy Mummy Food Company and developing The Make More Milk Method, Kelly is here to help you not only overcome low milk supply but also bid farewell to the challenges that often accompany motherhood – brain fog, exhaustion, and restless nights.

Her mission? To help you become the best version of yourself – the radiant, nourished mum your child, family, and community deserve.
In a world that's rapidly evolving, Kelly recognizes that the postpartum period is no longer about snapping back into your pre-baby body or being a superhero mom. It's about honoring the mother, nurturing her, and providing the nourishment she needs to heal, bond with her baby & in turn breastfeed with more ease & confidence.

Kelly xoxo

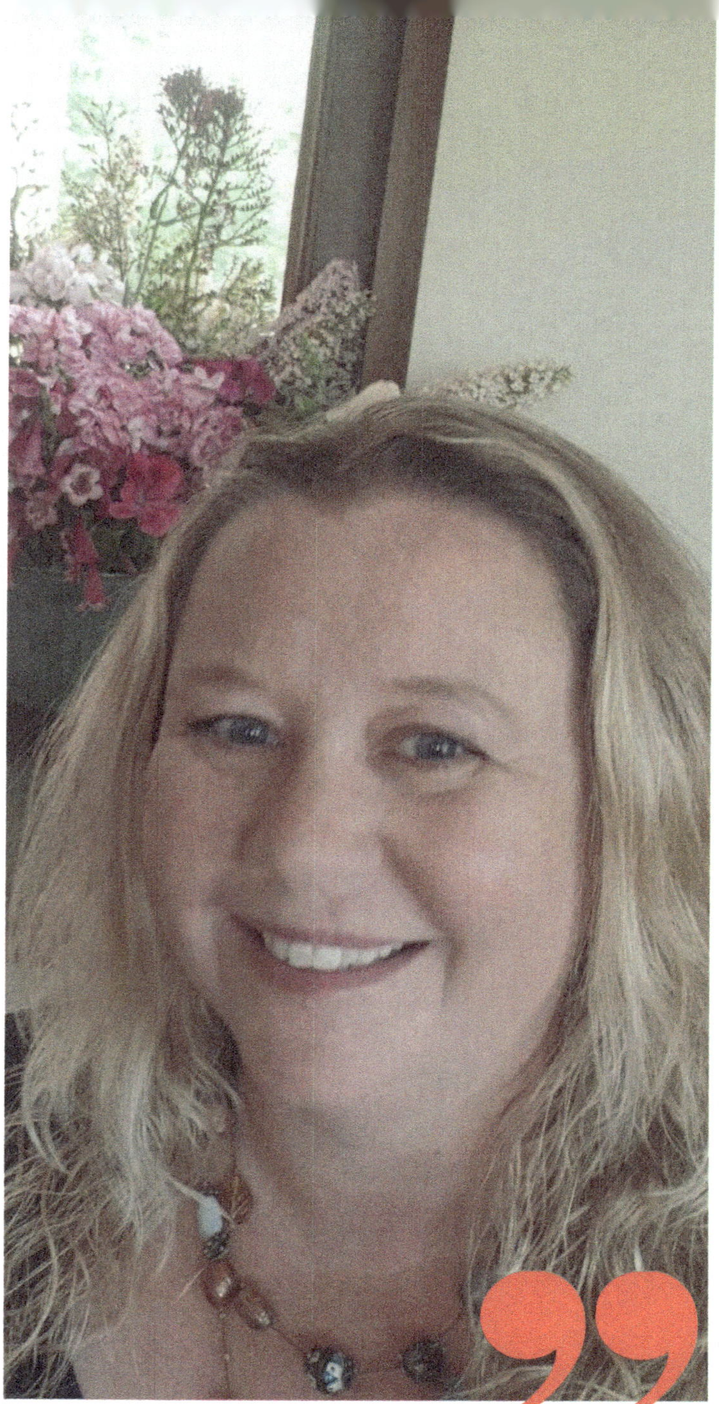

My mission is to help you overcome nutrient depletion, so you can increase your milk supply but also see other long term health and wellbeing benefits from this around postpartum healing including reduced brain fog, fatigue and even lessen postpartum mood disorders!

Introduction

Going through pregnancy and childbirth can feel like a whirlwind of changes. Suddenly, your body starts acting in ways you didn't expect, which can feel overwhelming. It's like you're on a road with many twists and turns without a map.

That's where the "Postpartum Essentials Breastfeeding Nutrition Daily Food & Reflection Diary" comes in. It's a guide to help you through this journey, and the main goal is for you to understand what's happening with your body.

Particularly how your dietary choices impact your feelings, mood, symptoms and even your milk supply!

It's like having a conversation and a deeper connection with your body. You'll notice that some foods might make you feel better, while others might trigger discomfort.

This diary is your space to jot down your meals, symptoms, and thoughts, while at the same time tracking your baby's feeding schedule or pumping schedule if you're pumping or mixed feeding.
Over time, you'll start seeing patterns, to help you learn what makes you feel good and what doesn't and what is helping to fuel your body for motherhood. It's all about getting to know your body better.

Plus, this diary can be a big help when you're working with a qualified professional, making it easier for them to help you through this transition.

It can also be a helpful tool to take with you when you visit your doctor or healthcare provider. It gives your healthcare professional a clear picture of what you've been experiencing.

The "Postpartum Essentials Breastfeeding Nutrition Daily Food & Reflection Diary" is a simple tool but can make a big difference. It's about taking small steps to understand and care for yourself better during your postpartum period. So, as you jot down a few notes each day, you're not just writing; you're taking control, learning, and making this journey a bit easier for yourself.

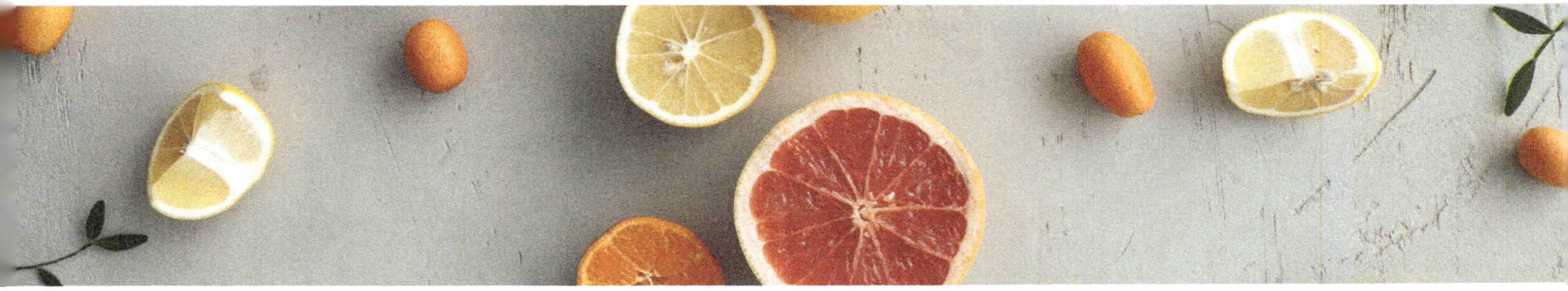

Benefits of keeping a Food & Reflection Diary

① Getting to Know Your Food

Food can change how you feel. This diary helps you keep an eye on what you eat and notice which foods make you feel good and which don't.

② Finding Patterns

You might start to see patterns when you write down your symptoms and what you eat. For example, you might find that certain foods stomach upsets or mood swings, and you can change your diet to feel better.

③ A Quiet Moment

Taking a little time to reflect on your day and jot down your thoughts can be calming. It's a moment for you and might help you feel more in control.

④ Learning About Yourself

Over time, you'll learn a lot about how your body reacts to different foods and situations. It's like getting to know yourself better.

⑤ Talking to Your Doctor or Healthcare Provider

When you visit your doctor or healthcare provider, having this diary can help you explain what's been going on, making it easier for them to understand and help you.

Your Concerns:

Is It Too Much Work?

- It might seem like a task to fill out a diary every day, but it's for a good reason - ***your well-being***. And once you get used to it, it'll only take a few minutes.

Will It Really Help?

- You might wonder if a diary can make a difference. It's a simple tool, but it can give powerful insights to help you navigate your postpartum period of time more comfortably.

Is Change Scary?

- Trying something new can be a bit scary, but small steps like keeping a daily diary can lead to big positive changes in how you feel.

Evening Reflections - Declutter Your Mind

As the day winds down, it's the perfect time to clear your mind. ***The Evening Reflections section lets you let go of the day's stresses,*** jot down your thoughts, and prepare for a peaceful night's sleep. It's like having a quiet conversation with yourself, which can be soothing and help you wake up refreshed and ready for the new day.

Let's get started...

1 WEEK First Steps

Day 1

BREAKFAST

LUNCH

DINNER

SNACKS

DRINKS CONSUMED *(INCLUDING ALCOHOL)*

SUPPLEMENTS/MEDICATIONS TAKEN

HUNGER LEVELS BEFORE EATING

○ ○ ○ ○ ○ ○ ○ ○ ○ ○

1- NOT HUNGRY *10 - RAVENOUS*

MOOD BEFORE EATING

○ ○ ○ ○ ○

MOOD 1 HR AFTER EATING

○ ○ ○ ○ ○

MOOD 3 HRS AFTER EATING

○ ○ ○ ○ ○

BREAKFAST

LUNCH

DINNER

SNACKS

DRINKS CONSUMED *(INCLUDING ALCOHOL)*

SUPPLEMENTS/MEDICATIONS TAKEN

HUNGER LEVELS BEFORE EATING

○ ○ ○ ○ ○ ○ ○ ○ ○ ○

1- NOT HUNGRY *10 - RAVENOUS*

MOOD BEFORE EATING

○ ○ ○ ○ ○

MOOD 1 HR AFTER EATING

○ ○ ○ ○ ○

MOOD 3 HRS AFTER EATING

○ ○ ○ ○ ○

1 WEEK

First Steps

Day 1

BREAKFAST

LUNCH

DINNER

SNACKS

DRINKS CONSUMED *(INCLUDING ALCOHOL)*

SUPPLEMENTS/MEDICATIONS TAKEN

HUNGER LEVELS BEFORE EATING

○ ○ ○ ○ ○ ○ ○ ○ ○ ○

1- NOT HUNGRY *10 - RAVENOUS*

MOOD BEFORE EATING

○ ○ ○ ○ ○

MOOD 1 HR AFTER EATING

○ ○ ○ ○ ○

MOOD 3 HRS AFTER EATING

○ ○ ○ ○ ○

BREAKFAST

LUNCH

DINNER

SNACKS

DRINKS CONSUMED *(INCLUDING ALCOHOL)*

SUPPLEMENTS/MEDICATIONS TAKEN

HUNGER LEVELS BEFORE EATING

○ ○ ○ ○ ○ ○ ○ ○ ○ ○

1- NOT HUNGRY *10 - RAVENOUS*

MOOD BEFORE EATING

○ ○ ○ ○ ○

MOOD 1 HR AFTER EATING

○ ○ ○ ○ ○

MOOD 3 HRS AFTER EATING

○ ○ ○ ○ ○

1 WEEK First Steps

Observations

____

____

____

____

____

____

- [ ] Bloating
- [ ] Energy Spike
- [ ] Irritability
- [ ] Headache
- [ ] Skin Reaction
- [ ] Nausea
- [ ] Vomiting
- [ ] Constipation
- [ ] Diarrhea
- [ ] Gas
- [ ] Other *(space for them to explain)*

____

Postpartum Symptoms

Symptoms Experienced

- [ ] Hot Flashes
- [ ] Sweating
- [ ] Night Sweats
- [ ] Anxiety
- [ ] Bloating
- [ ] Fatigue
- [ ] Gas
- [ ] Brain Fog
- [ ] Poor Concentration
- [ ] Mood Swings
- [ ] Cravings
- [ ] Sleep Disturbances
- [ ] Vaginal Dryness
- [ ] Headache
- [ ] Other (please explain)

____

- [ ] Mild
- [ ] Moderate
- [ ] Severe

Duration of Symptoms

____

____

____

____

____

____

____

- [ ] 5 Mins
- [ ] 15 Mins
- [ ] 1 Hour

New Symptoms:

Please explain

____

____

____

____

Observations:

Please explain

____

____

____

____

1 WEEK First Steps

Breastfeeding / Pumping Information

TIME	FEEDING / PUMPING		SLEEP OR ACTIVITY	BABY TOILETING	
	DURATION (Feeding)	AMOUNT (Bottle/ Pump)		PEE	POOP

Feelings & Observations

1 WEEK

First Steps

Physical Activity

Type of Activity:

Duration:

Intensity:

☐ Low ☐ Moderate ☐ High

Sleep

Quality of Sleep:

☐ Excellent
☐ Poor
☐ Good
☐ Very Poor
☐ Fair

Hours Slept:

____

____

____

Support System:

Stress Management Techniques:

Water Intake Tracker:

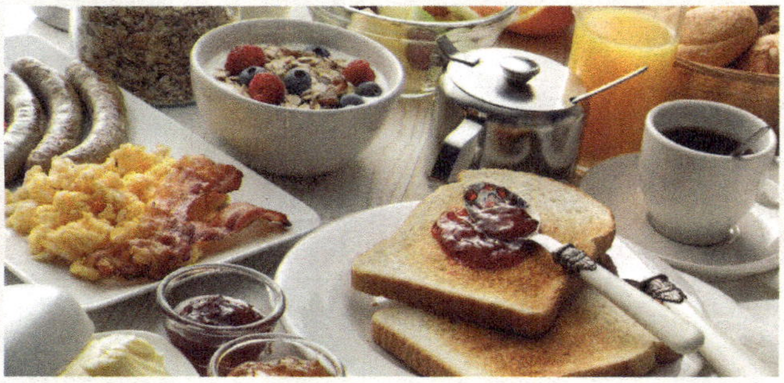

Overall Observations for the Day:

1
WEEK

Evening Reflections

Declutter Your Mind

As the day ends, take a moment to ***reflect on your day,*** and use this space to ***declutter your mind.*** Jot down your thoughts, feelings, and any moments that stood out. ***Often referred to as a "brain dump,"*** it's a method to understand, process, and release lingering thoughts that have built up throughout the day. Doing so will help to reduce stress and pave the way for a more peaceful night.

Thoughts/feelings

Use this space to let go of everything on your mind and write down your thoughts and feelings (from fleeting thoughts to deepest emotions). Writing them down without feeling "judged" helps you understand your feelings and prevents nighttime overthinking as you drift off to sleep.

Highlights and Today's Wins

What made you smile, feel proud, or brought you a sense of accomplishment today? Celebrate even the smallest wins and what you are especially thankful for here.

1
WEEK

Evening Reflections

Declutter Your Mind

Steps to Prepare For Tomorrow

Consider today's challenges. Which moments or areas is there room for growth or change? What steps can you take for a "better" tomorrow?

Rate Your Day

How would you describe your day on a scale of 1 to 10?
Use the emojis below as a guide, with 1 representing a difficult day and 10 symbolising an exceptional one...

1	2	3	4	5	6	7	8	9	10

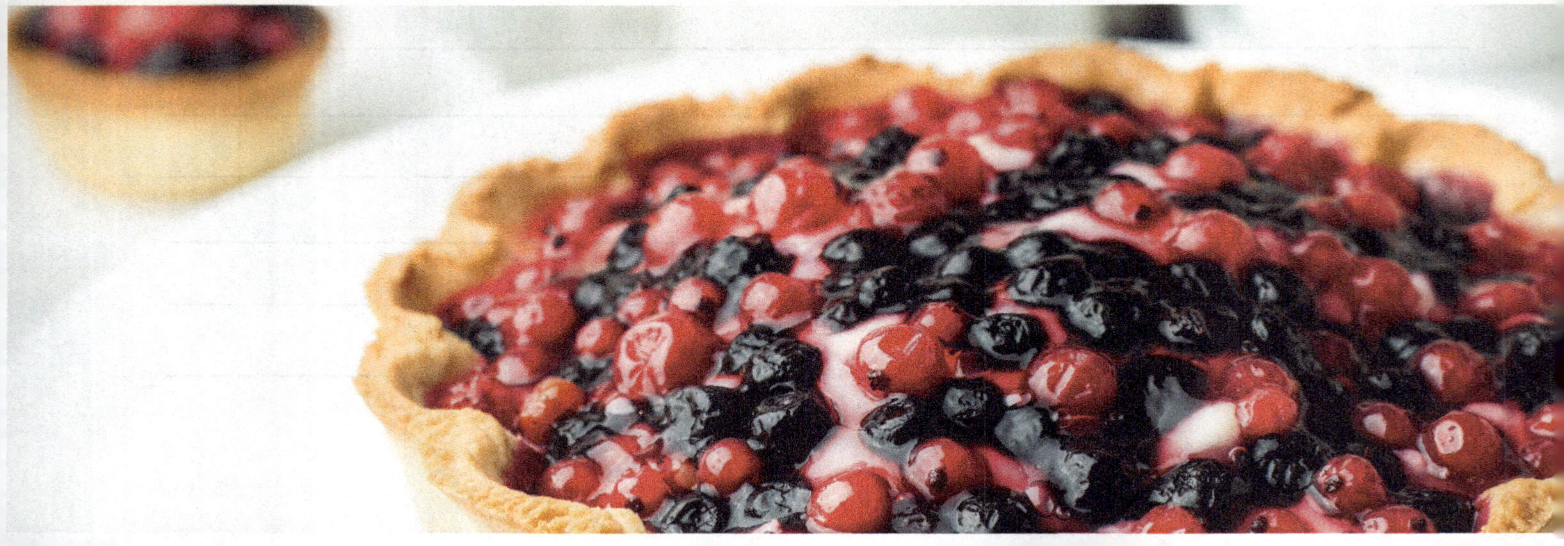

First Steps

Day 2

BREAKFAST

LUNCH

DINNER

SNACKS

DRINKS CONSUMED *(INCLUDING ALCOHOL)*

SUPPLEMENTS/MEDICATIONS TAKEN

HUNGER LEVELS BEFORE EATING

○ ○ ○ ○ ○ ○ ○ ○ ○ ○

1- NOT HUNGRY *10 - RAVENOUS*

MOOD BEFORE EATING

○ ○ ○ ○ ○

MOOD 1 HR AFTER EATING

○ ○ ○ ○ ○

MOOD 3 HRS AFTER EATING

○ ○ ○ ○ ○

BREAKFAST

LUNCH

DINNER

SNACKS

DRINKS CONSUMED *(INCLUDING ALCOHOL)*

SUPPLEMENTS/MEDICATIONS TAKEN

HUNGER LEVELS BEFORE EATING

○ ○ ○ ○ ○ ○ ○ ○ ○ ○

1- NOT HUNGRY *10 - RAVENOUS*

MOOD BEFORE EATING

○ ○ ○ ○ ○

MOOD 1 HR AFTER EATING

○ ○ ○ ○ ○

MOOD 3 HRS AFTER EATING

○ ○ ○ ○ ○

1 WEEK

First Steps

Day 2

BREAKFAST

LUNCH

DINNER

SNACKS

DRINKS CONSUMED *(INCLUDING ALCOHOL)*

SUPPLEMENTS/MEDICATIONS TAKEN

HUNGER LEVELS BEFORE EATING

○ ○ ○ ○ ○ ○ ○ ○ ○ ○

1- NOT HUNGRY *10 - RAVENOUS*

MOOD BEFORE EATING

○ ○ ○ ○ ○

MOOD 1 HR AFTER EATING

○ ○ ○ ○ ○

MOOD 3 HRS AFTER EATING

○ ○ ○ ○ ○

BREAKFAST

LUNCH

DINNER

SNACKS

DRINKS CONSUMED *(INCLUDING ALCOHOL)*

SUPPLEMENTS/MEDICATIONS TAKEN

HUNGER LEVELS BEFORE EATING

○ ○ ○ ○ ○ ○ ○ ○ ○ ○

1- NOT HUNGRY *10 - RAVENOUS*

MOOD BEFORE EATING

○ ○ ○ ○ ○

MOOD 1 HR AFTER EATING

○ ○ ○ ○ ○

MOOD 3 HRS AFTER EATING

○ ○ ○ ○ ○

1 WEEK First Steps

Observations

- [ ] Bloating
- [ ] Energy Spike
- [ ] Irritability
- [ ] Headache
- [ ] Skin Reaction
- [ ] Nausea
- [ ] Vomiting
- [ ] Constipation
- [ ] Diarrhea
- [ ] Gas
- [ ] Other *(space for them to explain)*

Perimenopausal/Menopausal Symptoms

Symptoms Experienced

- [ ] Hot Flashes
- [ ] Sweating
- [ ] Night Sweats
- [ ] Anxiety
- [ ] Bloating
- [ ] Fatigue
- [ ] Gas
- [ ] Brain Fog
- [ ] Poor Concentration
- [ ] Mood Swings
- [ ] Cravings
- [ ] Sleep Disturbances
- [ ] Vaginal Dryness
- [ ] Headache
- [ ] Other (please explain)

- [ ] Mild
- [ ] Moderate
- [ ] Severe

Duration of Symptoms

- [ ] 5 Mins
- [ ] 15 Mins
- [ ] 1 Hour

New Symptoms:
Please explain

Observations:
Please explain

1
WEEK

First Steps

Physical Activity

Type of Activity:

Duration:

Intensity:

- [ ] Low
- [ ] Moderate
- [ ] High

Sleep

Quality of Sleep:

- [ ] Excellent
- [ ] Poor
- [ ] Good
- [ ] Very Poor
- [ ] Fair

Hours Slept:

Support System:

Stress Management Techniques:

Water Intake Tracker:

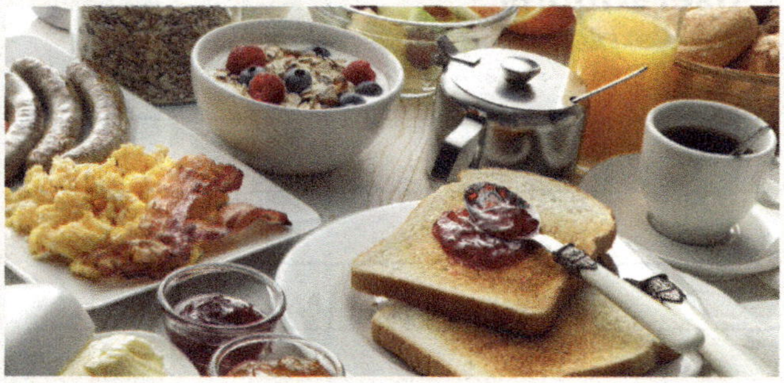

Overall Observations for the Day:

1 WEEK

Evening Reflections

Declutter Your Mind

As the day ends, take a moment to ***reflect on your day,*** and use this space to ***declutter your mind.*** Jot down your thoughts, feelings, and any moments that stood out. ***Often referred to as a "brain dump,"*** it's a method to understand, process, and release lingering thoughts that have built up throughout the day. Doing so will help to reduce stress and pave the way for a more peaceful night.

Thoughts/feelings

Use this space to let go of everything on your mind and write down your thoughts and feelings (from fleeting thoughts to deepest emotions). Writing them down without feeling "judged" helps you understand your feelings and prevents nighttime overthinking as you drift off to sleep.

Highlights and Today's Wins

What made you smile, feel proud, or brought you a sense of accomplishment today? Celebrate even the smallest wins and what you are especially thankful for here.

First Steps

Day 2

BREAKFAST

LUNCH

DINNER

SNACKS

DRINKS CONSUMED *(INCLUDING ALCOHOL)*

SUPPLEMENTS/MEDICATIONS TAKEN

HUNGER LEVELS BEFORE EATING

○ ○ ○ ○ ○ ○ ○ ○ ○ ○

1- NOT HUNGRY *10 - RAVENOUS*

MOOD BEFORE EATING

○ ○ ○ ○ ○

MOOD 1 HR AFTER EATING

○ ○ ○ ○ ○

MOOD 3 HRS AFTER EATING

○ ○ ○ ○ ○

BREAKFAST

LUNCH

DINNER

SNACKS

DRINKS CONSUMED *(INCLUDING ALCOHOL)*

SUPPLEMENTS/MEDICATIONS TAKEN

HUNGER LEVELS BEFORE EATING

○ ○ ○ ○ ○ ○ ○ ○ ○ ○

1- NOT HUNGRY *10 - RAVENOUS*

MOOD BEFORE EATING

○ ○ ○ ○ ○

MOOD 1 HR AFTER EATING

○ ○ ○ ○ ○

MOOD 3 HRS AFTER EATING

○ ○ ○ ○ ○

BREAKFAST

LUNCH

DINNER

SNACKS

DRINKS CONSUMED *(INCLUDING ALCOHOL)*

SUPPLEMENTS/MEDICATIONS TAKEN

HUNGER LEVELS BEFORE EATING

○ ○ ○ ○ ○ ○ ○ ○ ○ ○

1- NOT HUNGRY *10 - RAVENOUS*

MOOD BEFORE EATING

○ ○ ○ ○ ○

MOOD 1 HR AFTER EATING

○ ○ ○ ○ ○

MOOD 3 HRS AFTER EATING

○ ○ ○ ○ ○

BREAKFAST

LUNCH

DINNER

SNACKS

DRINKS CONSUMED *(INCLUDING ALCOHOL)*

SUPPLEMENTS/MEDICATIONS TAKEN

HUNGER LEVELS BEFORE EATING

○ ○ ○ ○ ○ ○ ○ ○ ○ ○

1- NOT HUNGRY *10 - RAVENOUS*

MOOD BEFORE EATING

○ ○ ○ ○ ○

MOOD 1 HR AFTER EATING

○ ○ ○ ○ ○

MOOD 3 HRS AFTER EATING

○ ○ ○ ○ ○

1 WEEK First Steps

Observations

- [ ] Bloating
- [ ] Energy Spike
- [ ] Irritability
- [ ] Headache
- [ ] Skin Reaction
- [ ] Nausea
- [ ] Vomiting
- [ ] Constipation
- [ ] Diarrhea
- [ ] Gas
- [ ] Other *(space for them to explain)*

Perimenopausal/Menopausal Symptoms

Symptoms Experienced

- [ ] Hot Flashes
- [ ] Sweating
- [ ] Night Sweats
- [ ] Anxiety
- [ ] Bloating
- [ ] Fatigue
- [ ] Gas
- [ ] Brain Fog
- [ ] Poor Concentration
- [ ] Mood Swings
- [ ] Cravings
- [ ] Sleep Disturbances
- [ ] Vaginal Dryness
- [ ] Headache
- [ ] Other (please explain)

- [ ] Mild
- [ ] Moderate
- [ ] Severe

Duration of Symptoms

- [ ] 5 Mins
- [ ] 15 Mins
- [ ] 1 Hour

New Symptoms:
Please explain

Observations:
Please explain

1 WEEK

First Steps

Breastfeeding / Pumping Information

TIME	FEEDING / PUMPING		SLEEP OR ACTIVITY	BABY TOILETING	
	DURATION (Feeding)	AMOUNT (Bottle/ Pump)		PEE	POOP

Feelings & Observations

1
WEEK

First Steps

Physical Activity

Type of Activity:

Duration:

Intensity:

☐ Low ☐ Moderate ☐ High

Sleep

Quality of Sleep:

☐ Excellent
☐ Good
☐ Fair
☐ Poor
☐ Very Poor

Hours Slept:

____

____

____

Support System:

Stress Management Techniques:

Water Intake Tracker:

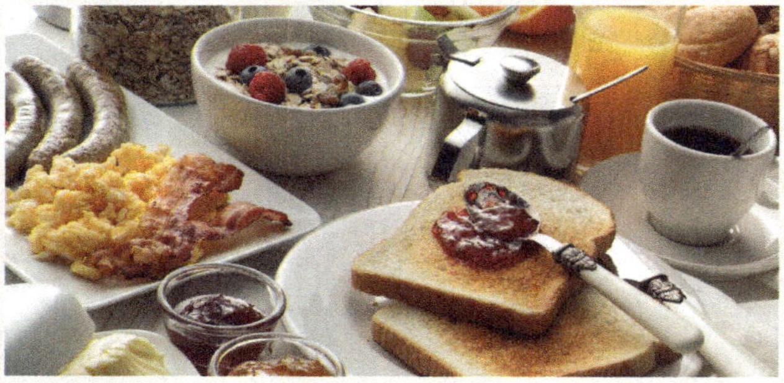

Overall Observations for the Day:

1 WEEK

Evening Reflections

Declutter Your Mind

As the day ends, take a moment to ***reflect on your day,*** and use this space to ***declutter your mind.*** Jot down your thoughts, feelings, and any moments that stood out. ***Often referred to as a "brain dump,"*** it's a method to understand, process, and release lingering thoughts that have built up throughout the day. Doing so will help to reduce stress and pave the way for a more peaceful night.

Thoughts/feelings

Use this space to let go of everything on your mind and write down your thoughts and feelings (from fleeting thoughts to deepest emotions). Writing them down without feeling "judged" helps you understand your feelings and prevents nighttime overthinking as you drift off to sleep.

Highlights and Today's Wins

What made you smile, feel proud, or brought you a sense of accomplishment today? Celebrate even the smallest wins and what you are especially thankful for here.

1 WEEK Evening Reflections

Declutter Your Mind

Steps to Prepare For Tomorrow

Consider today's challenges. Which moments or areas is there room for growth or change? What steps can you take for a "better" tomorrow?

Rate Your Day

How would you describe your day on a scale of 1 to 10?
Use the emojis below as a guide, with 1 representing a difficult day and 10 symbolising an exceptional one...

1	2	3	4	5	6	7	8	9	10

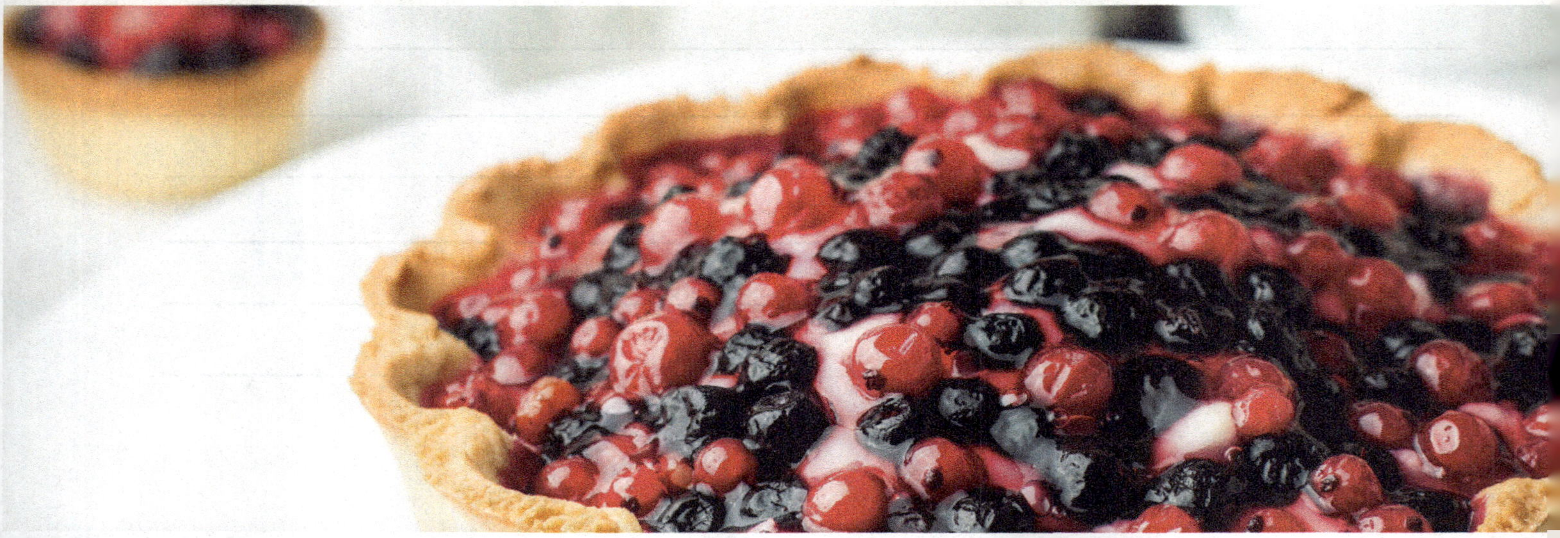

First Steps

Day 3

BREAKFAST

LUNCH

DINNER

SNACKS

DRINKS CONSUMED *(INCLUDING ALCOHOL)*

SUPPLEMENTS/MEDICATIONS TAKEN

HUNGER LEVELS BEFORE EATING

○ ○ ○ ○ ○ ○ ○ ○ ○ ○

1- NOT HUNGRY *10 - RAVENOUS*

MOOD BEFORE EATING

○ ○ ○ ○ ○

MOOD 1 HR AFTER EATING

○ ○ ○ ○ ○

MOOD 3 HRS AFTER EATING

○ ○ ○ ○ ○

BREAKFAST

LUNCH

DINNER

SNACKS

DRINKS CONSUMED *(INCLUDING ALCOHOL)*

SUPPLEMENTS/MEDICATIONS TAKEN

HUNGER LEVELS BEFORE EATING

○ ○ ○ ○ ○ ○ ○ ○ ○ ○

1- NOT HUNGRY *10 - RAVENOUS*

MOOD BEFORE EATING

○ ○ ○ ○ ○

MOOD 1 HR AFTER EATING

○ ○ ○ ○ ○

MOOD 3 HRS AFTER EATING

○ ○ ○ ○ ○

1 WEEK

First Steps

Day 3

BREAKFAST

LUNCH

DINNER

SNACKS

DRINKS CONSUMED *(INCLUDING ALCOHOL)*

SUPPLEMENTS/MEDICATIONS TAKEN

HUNGER LEVELS BEFORE EATING

○ ○ ○ ○ ○ ○ ○ ○ ○ ○

1- NOT HUNGRY *10 - RAVENOUS*

MOOD BEFORE EATING

○ ○ ○ ○ ○

MOOD 1 HR AFTER EATING

○ ○ ○ ○ ○

MOOD 3 HRS AFTER EATING

○ ○ ○ ○ ○

BREAKFAST

LUNCH

DINNER

SNACKS

DRINKS CONSUMED *(INCLUDING ALCOHOL)*

SUPPLEMENTS/MEDICATIONS TAKEN

HUNGER LEVELS BEFORE EATING

○ ○ ○ ○ ○ ○ ○ ○ ○ ○

1- NOT HUNGRY *10 - RAVENOUS*

MOOD BEFORE EATING

○ ○ ○ ○ ○

MOOD 1 HR AFTER EATING

○ ○ ○ ○ ○

MOOD 3 HRS AFTER EATING

○ ○ ○ ○ ○

1 WEEK First Steps

Observations

☐ Bloating
☐ Energy Spike
☐ Irritability
☐ Headache
☐ Skin Reaction
☐ Nausea
☐ Vomiting
☐ Constipation
☐ Diarrhea
☐ Gas
☐ Other *(space for them to explain)*

Perimenopausal/Menopausal Symptoms

Symptoms Experienced

☐ Hot Flashes
☐ Sweating
☐ Night Sweats
☐ Anxiety
☐ Bloating
☐ Fatigue
☐ Gas
☐ Brain Fog
☐ Poor Concentration
☐ Mood Swings
☐ Cravings
☐ Sleep Disturbances
☐ Vaginal Dryness
☐ Headache
☐ Other (please explain)

☐ Mild ☐ Moderate ☐ Severe

Duration of Symptoms

☐ 5 Mins ☐ 15 Mins ☐ 1 Hour

New Symptoms:
Please explain

Observations:
Please explain

1 WEEK

First Steps

Breastfeeding / Pumping Information

TIME	FEEDING / PUMPING		SLEEP OR ACTIVITY	BABY TOILETING	
	DURATION (Feeding)	AMOUNT (Bottle/ Pump)		PEE	POOP

Feelings & Observations

1 WEEK First Steps

Physical Activity

Type of Activity:

Duration:

Intensity:

- ☐ Low
- ☐ Moderate
- ☐ High

Sleep

Quality of Sleep:

- ☐ Excellent
- ☐ Poor
- ☐ Good
- ☐ Very Poor
- ☐ Fair

Hours Slept:

Support System:

Stress Management Techniques:

Water Intake Tracker:

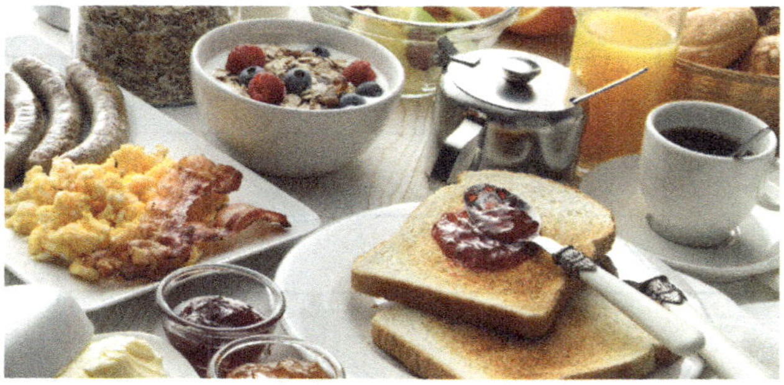

Overall Observations for the Day:

1 WEEK

Evening Reflections

Declutter Your Mind

As the day ends, take a moment to ***reflect on your day,*** and use this space to ***declutter your mind.*** Jot down your thoughts, feelings, and any moments that stood out. ***Often referred to as a "brain dump,"*** it's a method to understand, process, and release lingering thoughts that have built up throughout the day. Doing so will help to reduce stress and pave the way for a more peaceful night.

Thoughts/feelings

Use this space to let go of everything on your mind and write down your thoughts and feelings (from fleeting thoughts to deepest emotions). Writing them down without feeling "judged" helps you understand your feelings and prevents nighttime overthinking as you drift off to sleep.

Highlights and Today's Wins

What made you smile, feel proud, or brought you a sense of accomplishment today? Celebrate even the smallest wins and what you are especially thankful for here.

1 WEEK

Evening Reflections

Declutter Your Mind

Steps to Prepare For Tomorrow

Consider today's challenges. Which moments or areas is there room for growth or change? What steps can you take for a "better" tomorrow?

Rate Your Day

How would you describe your day on a scale of 1 to 10?
Use the emojis below as a guide, with 1 representing a difficult day and 10 symbolising an exceptional one...

1	2	3	4	5	6	7	8	9	10

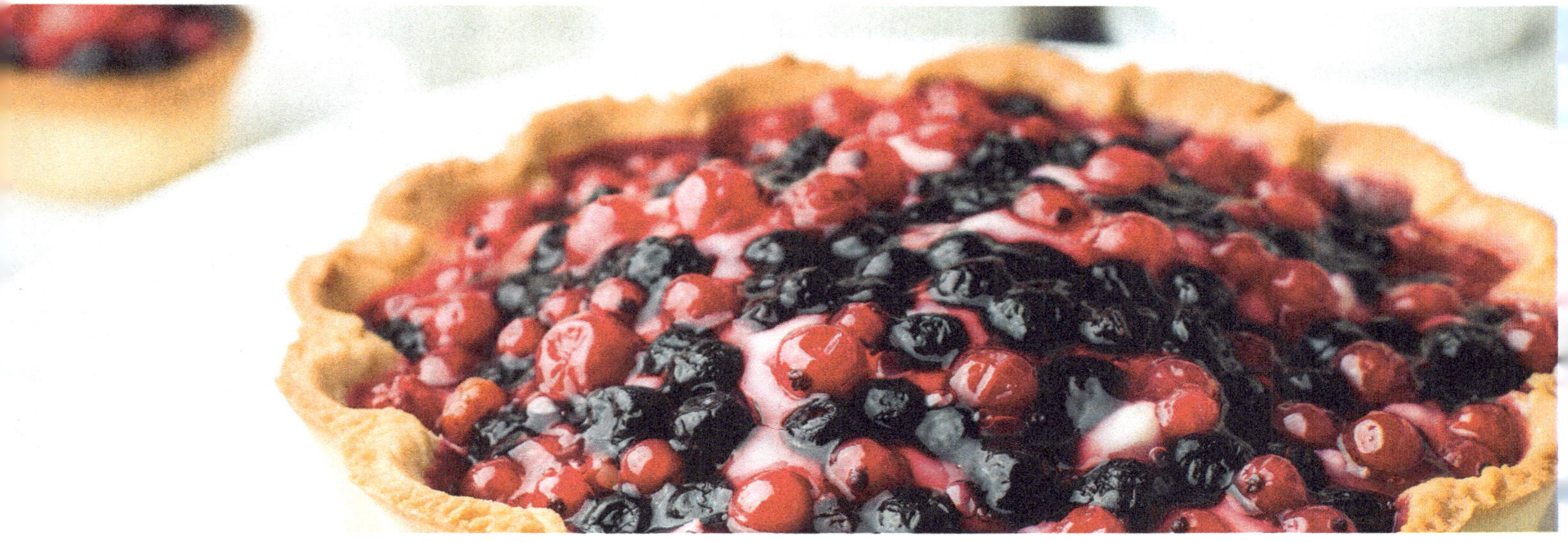

First Steps

Day 4

BREAKFAST

LUNCH

DINNER

SNACKS

DRINKS CONSUMED *(INCLUDING ALCOHOL)*

SUPPLEMENTS/MEDICATIONS TAKEN

HUNGER LEVELS BEFORE EATING

○ ○ ○ ○ ○ ○ ○ ○ ○ ○

1- NOT HUNGRY *10 - RAVENOUS*

MOOD BEFORE EATING

○ ○ ○ ○ ○

MOOD 1 HR AFTER EATING

○ ○ ○ ○ ○

MOOD 3 HRS AFTER EATING

○ ○ ○ ○ ○

BREAKFAST

LUNCH

DINNER

SNACKS

DRINKS CONSUMED *(INCLUDING ALCOHOL)*

SUPPLEMENTS/MEDICATIONS TAKEN

HUNGER LEVELS BEFORE EATING

○ ○ ○ ○ ○ ○ ○ ○ ○ ○

1- NOT HUNGRY *10 - RAVENOUS*

MOOD BEFORE EATING

○ ○ ○ ○ ○

MOOD 1 HR AFTER EATING

○ ○ ○ ○ ○

MOOD 3 HRS AFTER EATING

○ ○ ○ ○ ○

First Steps

Day 4

BREAKFAST

LUNCH

DINNER

SNACKS

DRINKS CONSUMED *(INCLUDING ALCOHOL)*

SUPPLEMENTS/MEDICATIONS TAKEN

HUNGER LEVELS BEFORE EATING

○ ○ ○ ○ ○ ○ ○ ○ ○ ○

1- NOT HUNGRY *10 - RAVENOUS*

MOOD BEFORE EATING

○ ○ ○ ○ ○

MOOD 1 HR AFTER EATING

○ ○ ○ ○ ○

MOOD 3 HRS AFTER EATING

○ ○ ○ ○ ○

BREAKFAST

LUNCH

DINNER

SNACKS

DRINKS CONSUMED *(INCLUDING ALCOHOL)*

SUPPLEMENTS/MEDICATIONS TAKEN

HUNGER LEVELS BEFORE EATING

○ ○ ○ ○ ○ ○ ○ ○ ○ ○

1- NOT HUNGRY *10 - RAVENOUS*

MOOD BEFORE EATING

○ ○ ○ ○ ○

MOOD 1 HR AFTER EATING

○ ○ ○ ○ ○

MOOD 3 HRS AFTER EATING

○ ○ ○ ○ ○

1 WEEK

First Steps

Observations

- [ ] Bloating
- [ ] Energy Spike
- [ ] Irritability
- [ ] Headache
- [ ] Skin Reaction
- [ ] Nausea
- [ ] Vomiting
- [ ] Constipation
- [ ] Diarrhea
- [ ] Gas
- [ ] Other *(space for them to explain)*

Perimenopausal/Menopausal Symptoms

Symptoms Experienced

- [ ] Hot Flashes
- [ ] Sweating
- [ ] Night Sweats
- [ ] Anxiety
- [ ] Bloating
- [ ] Fatigue
- [ ] Gas
- [ ] Brain Fog
- [ ] Poor Concentration
- [ ] Mood Swings
- [ ] Cravings
- [ ] Sleep Disturbances
- [ ] Vaginal Dryness
- [ ] Headache
- [ ] Other (please explain)

- [ ] Mild
- [ ] Moderate
- [ ] Severe

Duration of Symptoms

- [ ] 5 Mins
- [ ] 15 Mins
- [ ] 1 Hour

New Symptoms:

Please explain

Observations:

Please explain

1 WEEK

First Steps

Breastfeeding / Pumping Information

TIME	FEEDING / PUMPING		SLEEP OR ACTIVITY	BABY TOILETING	
	DURATION (Feeding)	AMOUNT (Bottle/ Pump)		PEE	POOP

Feelings & Observations

1 WEEK First Steps

Physical Activity

Type of Activity:

Duration:

Intensity:
☐ Low ☐ Moderate ☐ High

Sleep

Quality of Sleep:
☐ Excellent ☐ Poor
☐ Good ☐ Very Poor
☐ Fair

Hours Slept:

___

___

___

Support System:

Stress Management Techniques:

Water Intake Tracker:

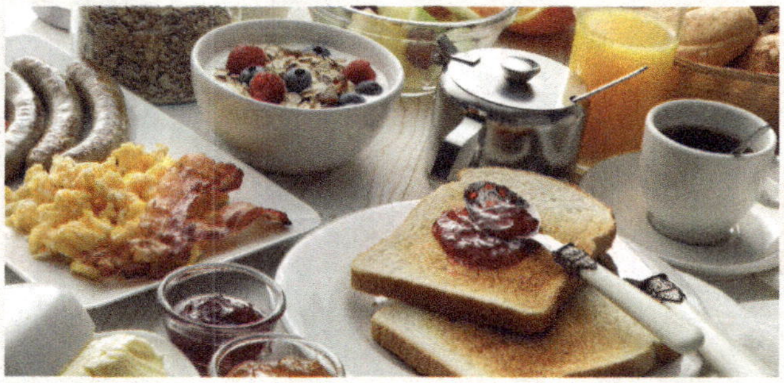

Overall Observations for the Day:

1 WEEK

Evening Reflections

Declutter Your Mind

As the day ends, take a moment to ***reflect on your day,*** and use this space to ***declutter your mind.*** Jot down your thoughts, feelings, and any moments that stood out. ***Often referred to as a "brain dump,"*** it's a method to understand, process, and release lingering thoughts that have built up throughout the day. Doing so will help to reduce stress and pave the way for a more peaceful night.

Thoughts/feelings

Use this space to let go of everything on your mind and write down your thoughts and feelings (from fleeting thoughts to deepest emotions). Writing them down without feeling "judged" helps you understand your feelings and prevents nighttime overthinking as you drift off to sleep.

Highlights and Today's Wins

What made you smile, feel proud, or brought you a sense of accomplishment today? Celebrate even the smallest wins and what you are especially thankful for here.

1 WEEK Evening Reflections

Declutter Your Mind

Steps to Prepare For Tomorrow

Consider today's challenges. Which moments or areas is there room for growth or change? What steps can you take for a "better" tomorrow?

Rate Your Day

How would you describe your day on a scale of 1 to 10?

Use the emojis below as a guide, with 1 representing a difficult day and 10 symbolising an exceptional one...

1	2	3	4	5	6	7	8	9	10

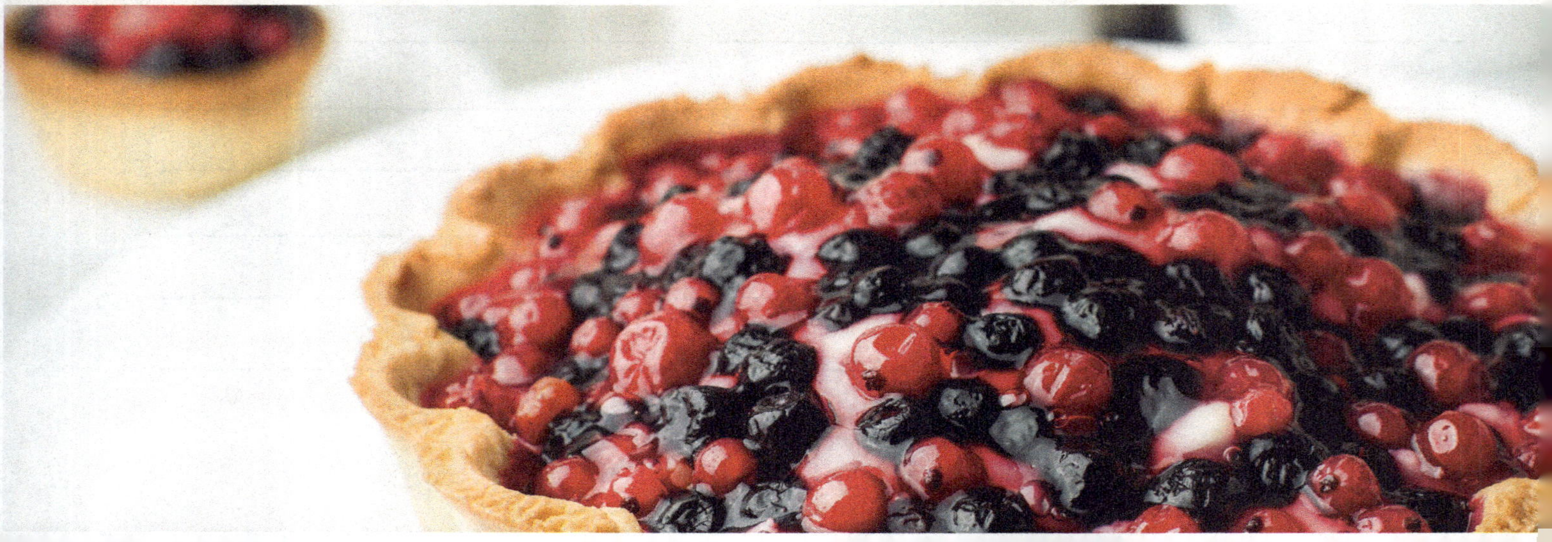

1 WEEK

First Steps

Day 5

BREAKFAST

LUNCH

DINNER

SNACKS

DRINKS CONSUMED *(INCLUDING ALCOHOL)*

SUPPLEMENTS/MEDICATIONS TAKEN

HUNGER LEVELS BEFORE EATING

○ ○ ○ ○ ○ ○ ○ ○ ○ ○

1- NOT HUNGRY *10 - RAVENOUS*

MOOD BEFORE EATING

○ ○ ○ ○ ○

MOOD 1 HR AFTER EATING

○ ○ ○ ○ ○

MOOD 3 HRS AFTER EATING

○ ○ ○ ○ ○

BREAKFAST

LUNCH

DINNER

SNACKS

DRINKS CONSUMED *(INCLUDING ALCOHOL)*

SUPPLEMENTS/MEDICATIONS TAKEN

HUNGER LEVELS BEFORE EATING

○ ○ ○ ○ ○ ○ ○ ○ ○ ○

1- NOT HUNGRY *10 - RAVENOUS*

MOOD BEFORE EATING

○ ○ ○ ○ ○

MOOD 1 HR AFTER EATING

○ ○ ○ ○ ○

MOOD 3 HRS AFTER EATING

○ ○ ○ ○ ○

First Steps

Day 5

BREAKFAST

LUNCH

DINNER

SNACKS

DRINKS CONSUMED *(INCLUDING ALCOHOL)*

SUPPLEMENTS/MEDICATIONS TAKEN

HUNGER LEVELS BEFORE EATING

○ ○ ○ ○ ○ ○ ○ ○ ○ ○

1- NOT HUNGRY *10 - RAVENOUS*

MOOD BEFORE EATING

○ ○ ○ ○ ○

MOOD 1 HR AFTER EATING

○ ○ ○ ○ ○

MOOD 3 HRS AFTER EATING

○ ○ ○ ○ ○

BREAKFAST

LUNCH

DINNER

SNACKS

DRINKS CONSUMED *(INCLUDING ALCOHOL)*

SUPPLEMENTS/MEDICATIONS TAKEN

HUNGER LEVELS BEFORE EATING

○ ○ ○ ○ ○ ○ ○ ○ ○ ○

1- NOT HUNGRY *10 - RAVENOUS*

MOOD BEFORE EATING

○ ○ ○ ○ ○

MOOD 1 HR AFTER EATING

○ ○ ○ ○ ○

MOOD 3 HRS AFTER EATING

○ ○ ○ ○ ○

1
WEEK

First Steps

Observations

- [ ] Bloating
- [ ] Energy Spike
- [ ] Irritability
- [ ] Headache
- [ ] Skin Reaction
- [ ] Nausea
- [ ] Vomiting
- [ ] Constipation
- [ ] Diarrhea
- [ ] Gas
- [ ] Other *(space for them to explain)*

Perimenopausal/Menopausal Symptoms

Symptoms Experienced

- [ ] Hot Flashes
- [ ] Sweating
- [ ] Night Sweats
- [ ] Anxiety
- [ ] Bloating
- [ ] Fatigue
- [ ] Gas
- [ ] Brain Fog
- [ ] Poor Concentration
- [ ] Mood Swings
- [ ] Cravings
- [ ] Sleep Disturbances
- [ ] Vaginal Dryness
- [ ] Headache
- [ ] Other (please explain)

- [ ] Mild
- [ ] Moderate
- [ ] Severe

Duration of Symptoms

- [ ] 5 Mins
- [ ] 15 Mins
- [ ] 1 Hour

New Symptoms:

Please explain

Observations:

Please explain

1 WEEK

First Steps

Breastfeeding / Pumping Information

TIME	FEEDING / PUMPING		SLEEP OR ACTIVITY	BABY TOILETING	
	DURATION (Feeding)	AMOUNT (Bottle/ Pump)		PEE	POOP

Feelings & Observations

1 WEEK

First Steps

Physical Activity

Type of Activity:

Duration:

Intensity:

- [ ] Low
- [ ] Moderate
- [ ] High

Sleep

Quality of Sleep:

- [ ] Excellent
- [ ] Poor
- [ ] Good
- [ ] Very Poor
- [ ] Fair

Hours Slept:

____

____

____

Support System:

Stress Management Techniques:

Water Intake Tracker:

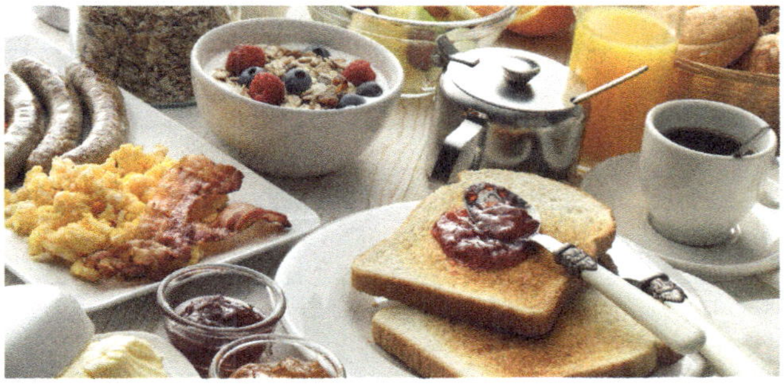

Overall Observations for the Day:

Evening Reflections

1 WEEK

Declutter Your Mind

As the day ends, take a moment to ***reflect on your day,*** and use this space to ***declutter your mind.*** Jot down your thoughts, feelings, and any moments that stood out. ***Often referred to as a "brain dump,"*** it's a method to understand, process, and release lingering thoughts that have built up throughout the day. Doing so will help to reduce stress and pave the way for a more peaceful night.

Thoughts/feelings

Use this space to let go of everything on your mind and write down your thoughts and feelings (from fleeting thoughts to deepest emotions). Writing them down without feeling "judged" helps you understand your feelings and prevents nighttime overthinking as you drift off to sleep.

Highlights and Today's Wins

What made you smile, feel proud, or brought you a sense of accomplishment today? Celebrate even the smallest wins and what you are especially thankful for here.

1 WEEK

Evening Reflections

Declutter Your Mind

Steps to Prepare For Tomorrow

Consider today's challenges. Which moments or areas is there room for growth or change? What steps can you take for a "better" tomorrow?

Rate Your Day

How would you describe your day on a scale of 1 to 10?
Use the emojis below as a guide, with 1 representing a difficult day and 10 symbolising an exceptional one...

1	2	3	4	5	6	7	8	9	10

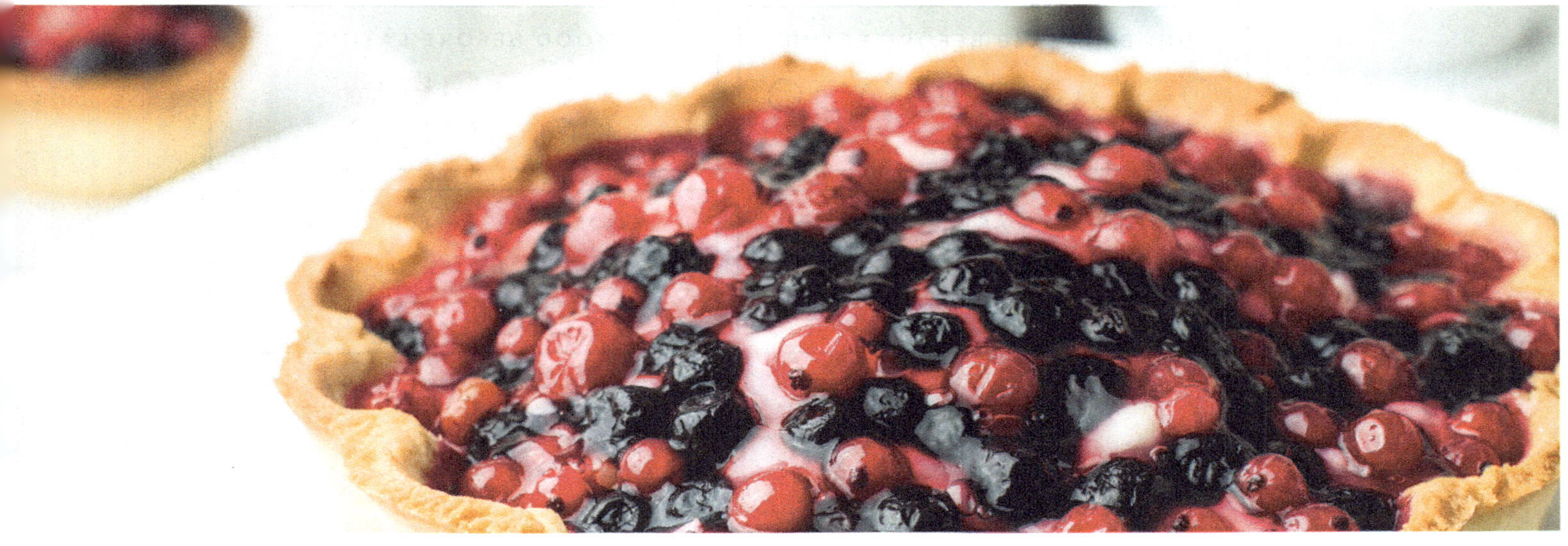

BREAKFAST

LUNCH

DINNER

SNACKS

DRINKS CONSUMED *(INCLUDING ALCOHOL)*

SUPPLEMENTS/MEDICATIONS TAKEN

HUNGER LEVELS BEFORE EATING

1- NOT HUNGRY *10 - RAVENOUS*

MOOD BEFORE EATING

MOOD 1 HR AFTER EATING

MOOD 3 HRS AFTER EATING

BREAKFAST

LUNCH

DINNER

SNACKS

DRINKS CONSUMED *(INCLUDING ALCOHOL)*

SUPPLEMENTS/MEDICATIONS TAKEN

HUNGER LEVELS BEFORE EATING

1- NOT HUNGRY *10 - RAVENOUS*

MOOD BEFORE EATING

MOOD 1 HR AFTER EATING

MOOD 3 HRS AFTER EATING

BREAKFAST

LUNCH

DINNER

SNACKS

DRINKS CONSUMED *(INCLUDING ALCOHOL)*

SUPPLEMENTS/MEDICATIONS TAKEN

HUNGER LEVELS BEFORE EATING

○ ○ ○ ○ ○ ○ ○ ○ ○ ○

1- NOT HUNGRY *10 - RAVENOUS*

MOOD BEFORE EATING

○ ○ ○ ○ ○

MOOD 1 HR AFTER EATING

○ ○ ○ ○ ○

MOOD 3 HRS AFTER EATING

○ ○ ○ ○ ○

BREAKFAST

LUNCH

DINNER

SNACKS

DRINKS CONSUMED *(INCLUDING ALCOHOL)*

SUPPLEMENTS/MEDICATIONS TAKEN

HUNGER LEVELS BEFORE EATING

○ ○ ○ ○ ○ ○ ○ ○ ○ ○

1- NOT HUNGRY *10 - RAVENOUS*

MOOD BEFORE EATING

○ ○ ○ ○ ○

MOOD 1 HR AFTER EATING

○ ○ ○ ○ ○

MOOD 3 HRS AFTER EATING

○ ○ ○ ○ ○

1 WEEK

First Steps

Observations

☐ Bloating
☐ Energy Spike
☐ Irritability
☐ Headache
☐ Skin Reaction
☐ Nausea
☐ Vomiting
☐ Constipation
☐ Diarrhea
☐ Gas
☐ Other *(space for them to explain)*

Perimenopausal/Menopausal Symptoms

Symptoms Experienced

☐ Hot Flashes
☐ Sweating
☐ Night Sweats
☐ Anxiety
☐ Bloating
☐ Fatigue
☐ Gas
☐ Brain Fog
☐ Poor Concentration
☐ Mood Swings
☐ Cravings
☐ Sleep Disturbances
☐ Vaginal Dryness
☐ Headache
☐ Other (please explain)

☐ Mild ☐ Moderate ☐ Severe

Duration of Symptoms

☐ 5 Mins ☐ 15 Mins ☐ 1 Hour

New Symptoms:

Please explain

Observations:

Please explain

1 WEEK First Steps

Physical Activity

Type of Activity:

Duration:

Intensity:

☐ Low ☐ Moderate ☐ High

Sleep

Quality of Sleep:

☐ Excellent ☐ Poor
☐ Good ☐ Very Poor
☐ Fair

Hours Slept:

Support System:

Stress Management Techniques:

Water Intake Tracker:

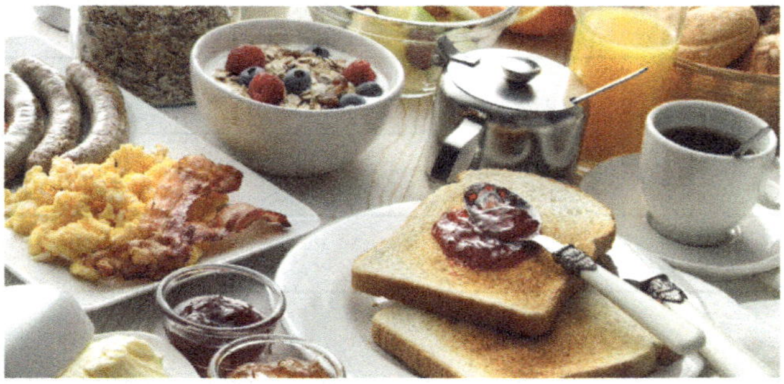

Overall Observations for the Day:

1
WEEK

Evening Reflections

Declutter Your Mind

As the day ends, take a moment to ***reflect on your day,*** and use this space to ***declutter your mind.*** Jot down your thoughts, feelings, and any moments that stood out. ***Often referred to as a "brain dump,"*** it's a method to understand, process, and release lingering thoughts that have built up throughout the day. Doing so will help to reduce stress and pave the way for a more peaceful night.

Thoughts/feelings

Use this space to let go of everything on your mind and write down your thoughts and feelings (from fleeting thoughts to deepest emotions). Writing them down without feeling "judged" helps you understand your feelings and prevents nighttime overthinking as you drift off to sleep.

Highlights and Today's Wins

What made you smile, feel proud, or brought you a sense of accomplishment today? Celebrate even the smallest wins and what you are especially thankful for here.

1 WEEK

Evening Reflections

Declutter Your Mind

Steps to Prepare For Tomorrow

Consider today's challenges. Which moments or areas is there room for growth or change? What steps can you take for a "better" tomorrow?

Rate Your Day

How would you describe your day on a scale of 1 to 10?
Use the emojis below as a guide, with 1 representing a difficult day and 10 symbolising an exceptional one...

1	2	3	4	5	6	7	8	9	10

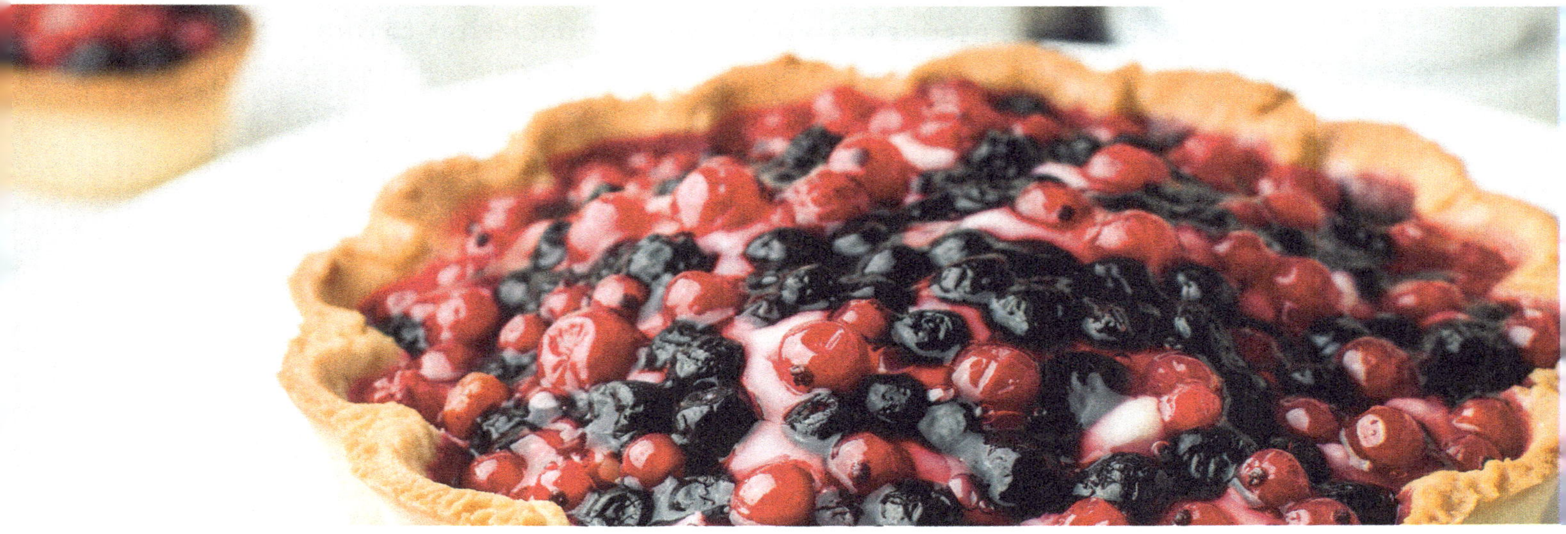

First Steps

Day 7

BREAKFAST

LUNCH

DINNER

SNACKS

DRINKS CONSUMED *(INCLUDING ALCOHOL)*

SUPPLEMENTS/MEDICATIONS TAKEN

HUNGER LEVELS BEFORE EATING

○ ○ ○ ○ ○ ○ ○ ○ ○ ○

1- NOT HUNGRY *10 - RAVENOUS*

MOOD BEFORE EATING

○ ○ ○ ○ ○

MOOD 1 HR AFTER EATING

○ ○ ○ ○ ○

MOOD 3 HRS AFTER EATING

○ ○ ○ ○ ○

BREAKFAST

LUNCH

DINNER

SNACKS

DRINKS CONSUMED *(INCLUDING ALCOHOL)*

SUPPLEMENTS/MEDICATIONS TAKEN

HUNGER LEVELS BEFORE EATING

○ ○ ○ ○ ○ ○ ○ ○ ○ ○

1- NOT HUNGRY *10 - RAVENOUS*

MOOD BEFORE EATING

○ ○ ○ ○ ○

MOOD 1 HR AFTER EATING

○ ○ ○ ○ ○

MOOD 3 HRS AFTER EATING

○ ○ ○ ○ ○

First Steps

Day 7

BREAKFAST

LUNCH

DINNER

SNACKS

DRINKS CONSUMED *(INCLUDING ALCOHOL)*

SUPPLEMENTS/MEDICATIONS TAKEN

HUNGER LEVELS BEFORE EATING

○ ○ ○ ○ ○ ○ ○ ○ ○ ○

1- NOT HUNGRY *10 - RAVENOUS*

MOOD BEFORE EATING

○ ○ ○ ○ ○

MOOD 1 HR AFTER EATING

○ ○ ○ ○ ○

MOOD 3 HRS AFTER EATING

○ ○ ○ ○ ○

BREAKFAST

LUNCH

DINNER

SNACKS

DRINKS CONSUMED *(INCLUDING ALCOHOL)*

SUPPLEMENTS/MEDICATIONS TAKEN

HUNGER LEVELS BEFORE EATING

○ ○ ○ ○ ○ ○ ○ ○ ○ ○

1- NOT HUNGRY *10 - RAVENOUS*

MOOD BEFORE EATING

○ ○ ○ ○ ○

MOOD 1 HR AFTER EATING

○ ○ ○ ○ ○

MOOD 3 HRS AFTER EATING

○ ○ ○ ○ ○

1 WEEK

First Steps

Observations

____

____

____

____

____

____

- ☐ Bloating
- ☐ Energy Spike
- ☐ Irritability
- ☐ Headache
- ☐ Skin Reaction
- ☐ Nausea
- ☐ Vomiting
- ☐ Constipation
- ☐ Diarrhea
- ☐ Gas
- ☐ Other *(space for them to explain)*

____

Perimenopausal/Menopausal Symptoms

Symptoms Experienced

- ☐ Hot Flashes
- ☐ Sweating
- ☐ Night Sweats
- ☐ Anxiety
- ☐ Bloating
- ☐ Fatigue
- ☐ Gas
- ☐ Brain Fog
- ☐ Poor Concentration
- ☐ Mood Swings
- ☐ Cravings
- ☐ Sleep Disturbances
- ☐ Vaginal Dryness
- ☐ Headache
- ☐ Other (please explain)

____

☐ Mild ☐ Moderate ☐ Severe

Duration of Symptoms

____

____

____

____

____

____

____

☐ 5 Mins ☐ 15 Mins ☐ 1 Hour

New Symptoms:

Please explain

____

____

____

____

Observations:

Please explain

____

____

____

____

1
WEEK

First Steps

Breastfeeding / Pumping Information

TIME	FEEDING / PUMPING		SLEEP OR ACTIVITY	BABY TOILETING	
	DURATION (Feeding)	AMOUNT (Bottle/ Pump)		PEE	POOP

Feelings & Observations

1 WEEK

First Steps

Physical Activity

Type of Activity:

Duration:

Intensity:

☐ Low ☐ Moderate ☐ High

Sleep

Quality of Sleep:

☐ Excellent ☐ Poor
☐ Good ☐ Very Poor
☐ Fair

Hours Slept:

____

____

____

Support System:

Stress Management Techniques:

Water Intake Tracker:

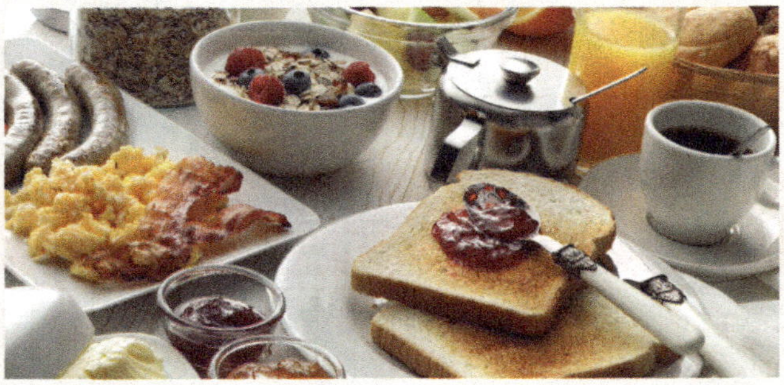

Overall Observations for the Day:

1
WEEK

Evening Reflections

Declutter Your Mind

As the day ends, take a moment to ***reflect on your day,*** and use this space to ***declutter your mind.*** Jot down your thoughts, feelings, and any moments that stood out. ***Often referred to as a "brain dump,"*** it's a method to understand, process, and release lingering thoughts that have built up throughout the day. Doing so will help to reduce stress and pave the way for a more peaceful night.

Thoughts/feelings

Use this space to let go of everything on your mind and write down your thoughts and feelings (from fleeting thoughts to deepest emotions). Writing them down without feeling "judged" helps you understand your feelings and prevents nighttime overthinking as you drift off to sleep.

Highlights and Today's Wins

What made you smile, feel proud, or brought you a sense of accomplishment today? Celebrate even the smallest wins and what you are especially thankful for here.

1
WEEK

Evening Reflections

Declutter Your Mind

Steps to Prepare For Tomorrow

Consider today's challenges. Which moments or areas is there room for growth or change? What steps can you take for a "better" tomorrow?

Rate Your Day

How would you describe your day on a scale of 1 to 10?
Use the emojis below as a guide, with 1 representing a difficult day and 10 symbolising an exceptional one...

1	2	3	4	5	6	7	8	9	10

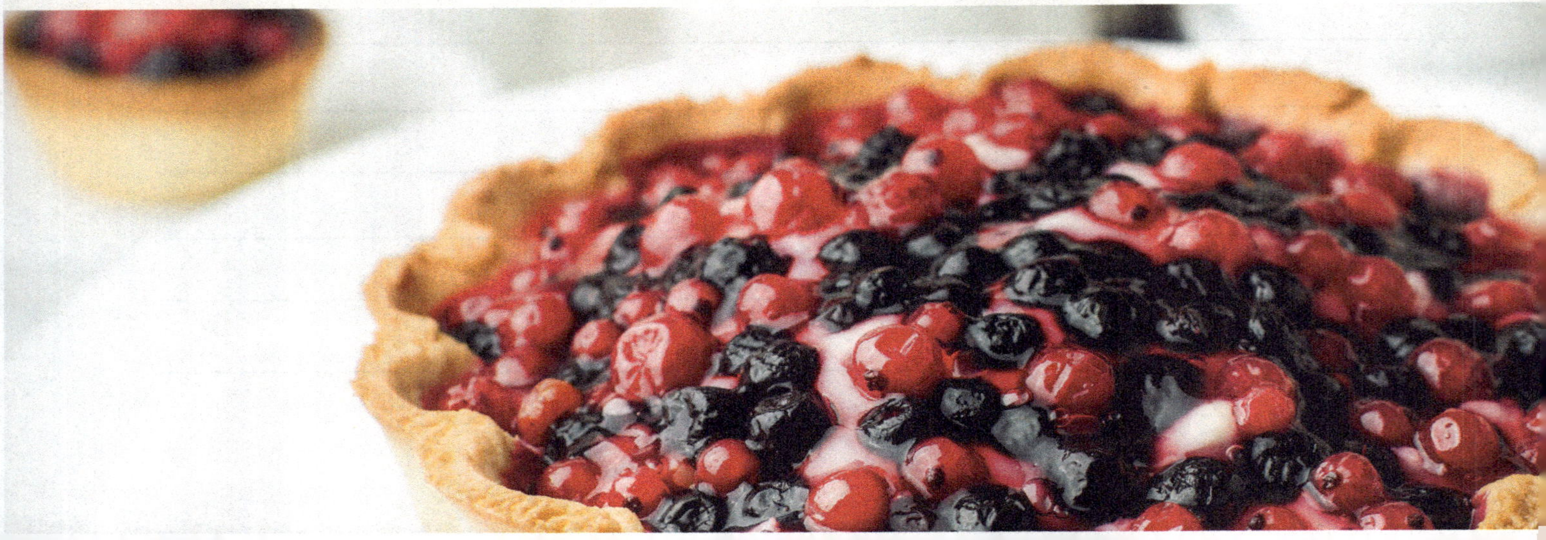

2 WEEK

Identifying Triggers

Day 1

Highlight any foods or drinks that seemed to worsen your symptoms during week one and monitor them closely during this week.

BREAKFAST

LUNCH

DINNER

SNACKS

DRINKS CONSUMED *(INCLUDING ALCOHOL)*

SUPPLEMENTS/MEDICATIONS TAKEN

HUNGER LEVELS BEFORE EATING

○ ○ ○ ○ ○ ○ ○ ○ ○ ○

1- NOT HUNGRY *10 - RAVENOUS*

MOOD BEFORE EATING

○ ○ ○ ○ ○

MOOD 1 HR AFTER EATING

○ ○ ○ ○ ○

MOOD 3 HRS AFTER EATING

○ ○ ○ ○ ○

BREAKFAST

LUNCH

DINNER

SNACKS

DRINKS CONSUMED *(INCLUDING ALCOHOL)*

SUPPLEMENTS/MEDICATIONS TAKEN

HUNGER LEVELS BEFORE EATING

○ ○ ○ ○ ○ ○ ○ ○ ○ ○

1- NOT HUNGRY *10 - RAVENOUS*

MOOD BEFORE EATING

○ ○ ○ ○ ○

MOOD 1 HR AFTER EATING

○ ○ ○ ○ ○

MOOD 3 HRS AFTER EATING

○ ○ ○ ○ ○

2
WEEK

Identifying Triggers

Day 1

Highlight any foods or drinks that seemed to worsen your symptoms during week one and monitor them closely during this week.

BREAKFAST

LUNCH

DINNER

SNACKS

DRINKS CONSUMED *(INCLUDING ALCOHOL)*

SUPPLEMENTS/MEDICATIONS TAKEN

HUNGER LEVELS BEFORE EATING

○ ○ ○ ○ ○ ○ ○ ○ ○ ○

1- NOT HUNGRY *10 - RAVENOUS*

MOOD BEFORE EATING

○ ○ ○ ○ ○

MOOD 1 HR AFTER EATING

○ ○ ○ ○ ○

MOOD 3 HRS AFTER EATING

○ ○ ○ ○ ○

BREAKFAST

LUNCH

DINNER

SNACKS

DRINKS CONSUMED *(INCLUDING ALCOHOL)*

SUPPLEMENTS/MEDICATIONS TAKEN

HUNGER LEVELS BEFORE EATING

○ ○ ○ ○ ○ ○ ○ ○ ○ ○

1- NOT HUNGRY *10 - RAVENOUS*

MOOD BEFORE EATING

○ ○ ○ ○ ○

MOOD 1 HR AFTER EATING

○ ○ ○ ○ ○

MOOD 3 HRS AFTER EATING

○ ○ ○ ○ ○

2
WEEK

Identifying Triggers

Highlight any foods or drinks that seemed to worsen your symptoms during week one and monitor them closely during this week.

Observations

____
____
____
____
____
____

- [ ] Bloating
- [ ] Nausea
- [ ] Energy Spike
- [ ] Vomiting
- [ ] Irritability
- [ ] Constipation
- [ ] Headache
- [ ] Diarrhea
- [ ] Skin Reaction
- [ ] Gas
- [ ] Other *(space for them to explain)*

____

Perimenopausal/Menopausal Symptoms

Symptoms Experienced

- [ ] Hot Flashes
- [ ] Poor Concentration
- [ ] Sweating
- [ ] Mood Swings
- [ ] Night Sweats
- [ ] Cravings
- [ ] Anxiety
- [ ] Sleep Disturbances
- [ ] Bloating
- [ ] Vaginal Dryness
- [ ] Fatigue
- [ ] Headache
- [ ] Gas
- [ ] Other (please explain)
- [ ] Brain Fog

____

- [ ] Mild
- [ ] Moderate
- [ ] Severe

Duration of Symptoms

____
____
____
____
____
____
____

- [ ] 5 Mins
- [ ] 15 Mins
- [ ] 1 Hour

New Symptoms:

Please explain

____
____
____
____

Observations:

Please explain

____
____
____
____

2 WEEK

Identifying Triggers

Breastfeeding / Pumping Information

TIME	FEEDING / PUMPING		SLEEP OR ACTIVITY	BABY TOILETING	
	DURATION (Feeding)	AMOUNT (Bottle/ Pump)		PEE	POOP

Feelings & Observations

2
WEEK

Evening Reflections

Declutter Your Mind

As the day ends, take a moment to ***reflect on your day,*** and use this space to ***declutter your mind.*** Jot down your thoughts, feelings, and any moments that stood out. ***Often referred to as a "brain dump,"*** it's a method to understand, process, and release lingering thoughts that have built up throughout the day. Doing so will help to reduce stress and pave the way for a more peaceful night.

Thoughts/feelings

Use this space to let go of everything on your mind and write down your thoughts and feelings (from fleeting thoughts to deepest emotions). Writing them down without feeling "judged" helps you understand your feelings and prevents nighttime overthinking as you drift off to sleep.

Highlights and Today's Wins

What made you smile, feel proud, or brought you a sense of accomplishment today? Celebrate even the smallest wins and what you are especially thankful for here.

2 WEEK

Evening Reflections

Declutter Your Mind

Steps to Prepare For Tomorrow

Consider today's challenges. Which moments or areas is there room for growth or change? What steps can you take for a "better" tomorrow?

Rate Your Day

How would you describe your day on a scale of 1 to 10?
Use the emojis below as a guide, with 1 representing a difficult day and 10 symbolising an exceptional one...

1	2	3	4	5	6	7	8	9	10

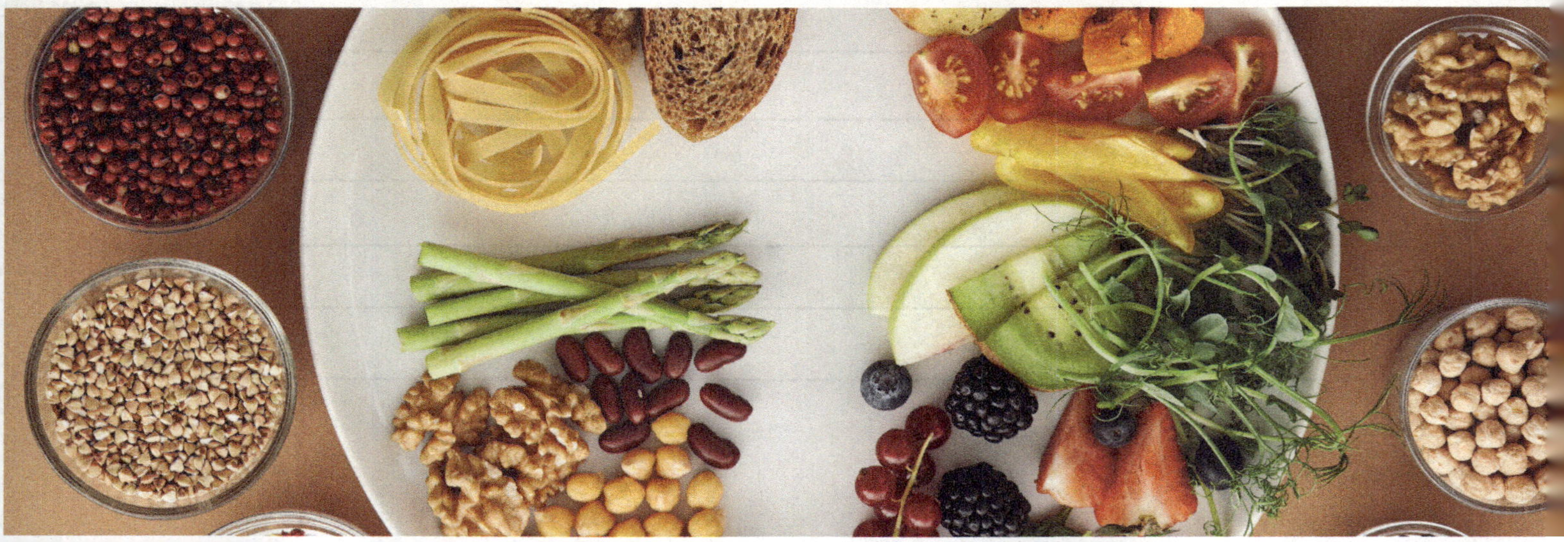

2 WEEK

Identifying Triggers

Day 2

Highlight any foods or drinks that seemed to worsen your symptoms during week one and monitor them closely during this week.

BREAKFAST

LUNCH

DINNER

SNACKS

DRINKS CONSUMED *(INCLUDING ALCOHOL)*

SUPPLEMENTS/MEDICATIONS TAKEN

HUNGER LEVELS BEFORE EATING

○ ○ ○ ○ ○ ○ ○ ○ ○ ○

1- NOT HUNGRY *10 - RAVENOUS*

MOOD BEFORE EATING

○ ○ ○ ○ ○

MOOD 1 HR AFTER EATING

○ ○ ○ ○ ○

MOOD 3 HRS AFTER EATING

○ ○ ○ ○ ○

BREAKFAST

LUNCH

DINNER

SNACKS

DRINKS CONSUMED *(INCLUDING ALCOHOL)*

SUPPLEMENTS/MEDICATIONS TAKEN

HUNGER LEVELS BEFORE EATING

○ ○ ○ ○ ○ ○ ○ ○ ○ ○

1- NOT HUNGRY *10 - RAVENOUS*

MOOD BEFORE EATING

○ ○ ○ ○ ○

MOOD 1 HR AFTER EATING

○ ○ ○ ○ ○

MOOD 3 HRS AFTER EATING

○ ○ ○ ○ ○

2 WEEK

Identifying Triggers

Day 2

Highlight any foods or drinks that seemed to worsen your symptoms during week one and monitor them closely during this week.

BREAKFAST

LUNCH

DINNER

SNACKS

DRINKS CONSUMED *(INCLUDING ALCOHOL)*

SUPPLEMENTS/MEDICATIONS TAKEN

HUNGER LEVELS BEFORE EATING

○ ○ ○ ○ ○ ○ ○ ○ ○ ○

1- NOT HUNGRY *10 - RAVENOUS*

MOOD BEFORE EATING

○ ○ ○ ○ ○

MOOD 1 HR AFTER EATING

○ ○ ○ ○ ○

MOOD 3 HRS AFTER EATING

○ ○ ○ ○ ○

BREAKFAST

LUNCH

DINNER

SNACKS

DRINKS CONSUMED *(INCLUDING ALCOHOL)*

SUPPLEMENTS/MEDICATIONS TAKEN

HUNGER LEVELS BEFORE EATING

○ ○ ○ ○ ○ ○ ○ ○ ○ ○

1- NOT HUNGRY *10 - RAVENOUS*

MOOD BEFORE EATING

○ ○ ○ ○ ○

MOOD 1 HR AFTER EATING

○ ○ ○ ○ ○

MOOD 3 HRS AFTER EATING

○ ○ ○ ○ ○

2 WEEK

Identifying Triggers

Highlight any foods or drinks that seemed to worsen your symptoms during week one and monitor them closely during this week.

Observations

____
____
____
____
____
____

- [ ] Bloating
- [ ] Nausea
- [ ] Energy Spike
- [ ] Vomiting
- [ ] Irritability
- [ ] Constipation
- [ ] Headache
- [ ] Diarrhea
- [ ] Skin Reaction
- [ ] Gas
- [ ] Other *(space for them to explain)*

____

Perimenopausal/Menopausal Symptoms

Symptoms Experienced

- [ ] Hot Flashes
- [ ] Poor Concentration
- [ ] Sweating
- [ ] Mood Swings
- [ ] Night Sweats
- [ ] Cravings
- [ ] Anxiety
- [ ] Sleep Disturbances
- [ ] Bloating
- [ ] Vaginal Dryness
- [ ] Fatigue
- [ ] Headache
- [ ] Gas
- [ ] Other (please explain)
- [ ] Brain Fog

____

- [ ] Mild
- [ ] Moderate
- [ ] Severe

Duration of Symptoms

____
____
____
____
____
____
____

- [ ] 5 Mins
- [ ] 15 Mins
- [ ] 1 Hour

New Symptoms:

Please explain

____
____
____
____

Observations:

Please explain

____
____
____
____

2 WEEK

Identifying Triggers

Breastfeeding / Pumping Information

TIME	FEEDING / PUMPING		SLEEP OR ACTIVITY	BABY TOILETING	
	DURATION (Feeding)	AMOUNT (Bottle/ Pump)		PEE	POOP

Feelings & Observations

2
WEEK

Evening Reflections

Declutter Your Mind

As the day ends, take a moment to ***reflect on your day,*** and use this space to ***declutter your mind.*** Jot down your thoughts, feelings, and any moments that stood out. ***Often referred to as a "brain dump,"*** it's a method to understand, process, and release lingering thoughts that have built up throughout the day. Doing so will help to reduce stress and pave the way for a more peaceful night.

Thoughts/feelings

Use this space to let go of everything on your mind and write down your thoughts and feelings (from fleeting thoughts to deepest emotions). Writing them down without feeling "judged" helps you understand your feelings and prevents nighttime overthinking as you drift off to sleep.

Highlights and Today's Wins

What made you smile, feel proud, or brought you a sense of accomplishment today? Celebrate even the smallest wins and what you are especially thankful for here.

2
WEEK

Evening Reflections

Declutter Your Mind

Steps to Prepare For Tomorrow

Consider today's challenges. Which moments or areas is there room for growth or change? What steps can you take for a "better" tomorrow?

Rate Your Day

How would you describe your day on a scale of 1 to 10?
Use the emojis below as a guide, with 1 representing a difficult day and 10 symbolising an exceptional one...

1	2	3	4	5	6	7	8	9	10

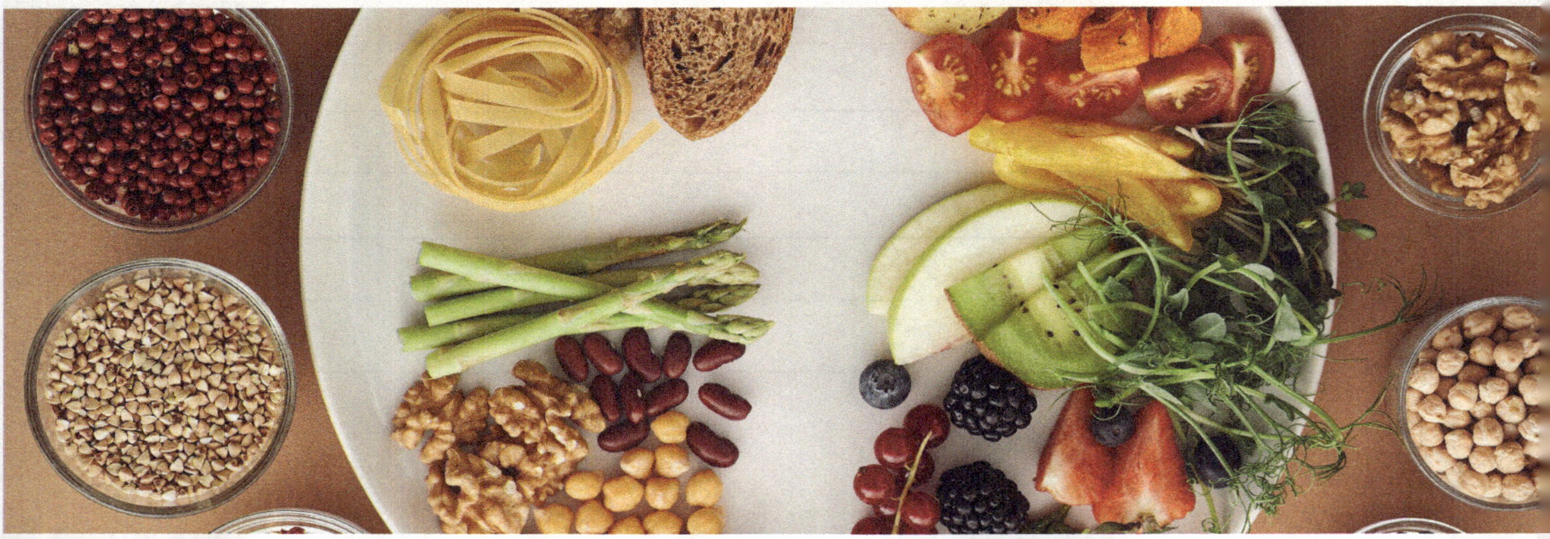

2
WEEK

Identifying Triggers

Day 3

Highlight any foods or drinks that seemed to worsen your symptoms during week one and monitor them closely during this week.

BREAKFAST

LUNCH

DINNER

SNACKS

DRINKS CONSUMED *(INCLUDING ALCOHOL)*

SUPPLEMENTS/MEDICATIONS TAKEN

HUNGER LEVELS BEFORE EATING

○ ○ ○ ○ ○ ○ ○ ○ ○ ○

1- NOT HUNGRY *10 - RAVENOUS*

MOOD BEFORE EATING

○ ○ ○ ○ ○

MOOD 1 HR AFTER EATING

○ ○ ○ ○ ○

MOOD 3 HRS AFTER EATING

○ ○ ○ ○ ○

BREAKFAST

LUNCH

DINNER

SNACKS

DRINKS CONSUMED *(INCLUDING ALCOHOL)*

SUPPLEMENTS/MEDICATIONS TAKEN

HUNGER LEVELS BEFORE EATING

○ ○ ○ ○ ○ ○ ○ ○ ○ ○

1- NOT HUNGRY *10 - RAVENOUS*

MOOD BEFORE EATING

○ ○ ○ ○ ○

MOOD 1 HR AFTER EATING

○ ○ ○ ○ ○

MOOD 3 HRS AFTER EATING

○ ○ ○ ○ ○

2
WEEK

Identifying Triggers

Day 3

Highlight any foods or drinks that seemed to worsen your symptoms during week one and monitor them closely during this week.

BREAKFAST

LUNCH

DINNER

SNACKS

DRINKS CONSUMED *(INCLUDING ALCOHOL)*

SUPPLEMENTS/MEDICATIONS TAKEN

HUNGER LEVELS BEFORE EATING

○ ○ ○ ○ ○ ○ ○ ○ ○ ○

1- NOT HUNGRY *10 - RAVENOUS*

MOOD BEFORE EATING

○ ○ ○ ○ ○

MOOD 1 HR AFTER EATING

○ ○ ○ ○ ○

MOOD 3 HRS AFTER EATING

○ ○ ○ ○ ○

BREAKFAST

LUNCH

DINNER

SNACKS

DRINKS CONSUMED *(INCLUDING ALCOHOL)*

SUPPLEMENTS/MEDICATIONS TAKEN

HUNGER LEVELS BEFORE EATING

○ ○ ○ ○ ○ ○ ○ ○ ○ ○

1- NOT HUNGRY *10 - RAVENOUS*

MOOD BEFORE EATING

○ ○ ○ ○ ○

MOOD 1 HR AFTER EATING

○ ○ ○ ○ ○

MOOD 3 HRS AFTER EATING

○ ○ ○ ○ ○

2 WEEK

Identifying Triggers

Day 3

Highlight any foods or drinks that seemed to worsen your symptoms during week one and monitor them closely during this week.

BREAKFAST

LUNCH

DINNER

SNACKS

DRINKS CONSUMED *(INCLUDING ALCOHOL)*

SUPPLEMENTS/MEDICATIONS TAKEN

HUNGER LEVELS BEFORE EATING

○ ○ ○ ○ ○ ○ ○ ○ ○ ○

1- NOT HUNGRY *10 - RAVENOUS*

MOOD BEFORE EATING

○ ○ ○ ○ ○

MOOD 1 HR AFTER EATING

○ ○ ○ ○ ○

MOOD 3 HRS AFTER EATING

○ ○ ○ ○ ○

BREAKFAST

LUNCH

DINNER

SNACKS

DRINKS CONSUMED *(INCLUDING ALCOHOL)*

SUPPLEMENTS/MEDICATIONS TAKEN

HUNGER LEVELS BEFORE EATING

○ ○ ○ ○ ○ ○ ○ ○ ○ ○

1- NOT HUNGRY *10 - RAVENOUS*

MOOD BEFORE EATING

○ ○ ○ ○ ○

MOOD 1 HR AFTER EATING

○ ○ ○ ○ ○

MOOD 3 HRS AFTER EATING

○ ○ ○ ○ ○

2
WEEK

Identifying Triggers

Highlight any foods or drinks that seemed to worsen your symptoms during week one and monitor them closely during this week.

Observations

____
____
____
____
____
____

- [ ] Bloating
- [ ] Energy Spike
- [ ] Irritability
- [ ] Headache
- [ ] Skin Reaction
- [ ] Nausea
- [ ] Vomiting
- [ ] Constipation
- [ ] Diarrhea
- [ ] Gas
- [ ] Other *(space for them to explain)*

____

Perimenopausal/Menopausal Symptoms

Symptoms Experienced

- [ ] Hot Flashes
- [ ] Sweating
- [ ] Night Sweats
- [ ] Anxiety
- [ ] Bloating
- [ ] Fatigue
- [ ] Gas
- [ ] Brain Fog
- [ ] Poor Concentration
- [ ] Mood Swings
- [ ] Cravings
- [ ] Sleep Disturbances
- [ ] Vaginal Dryness
- [ ] Headache
- [ ] Other (please explain)

____

- [ ] Mild
- [ ] Moderate
- [ ] Severe

Duration of Symptoms

____
____
____
____
____
____
____

- [ ] 5 Mins
- [ ] 15 Mins
- [ ] 1 Hour

New Symptoms:

Please explain

____
____
____
____

Observations:

Please explain

____
____
____
____

2 WEEK Identifying Triggers

Breastfeeding / Pumping Information

TIME	FEEDING / PUMPING		SLEEP OR ACTIVITY	BABY TOILETING	
	DURATION (Feeding)	AMOUNT (Bottle/ Pump)		PEE	POOP

Feelings & Observations

2
WEEK

Evening Reflections

Declutter Your Mind

As the day ends, take a moment to ***reflect on your day,*** and use this space to ***declutter your mind.*** Jot down your thoughts, feelings, and any moments that stood out. ***Often referred to as a "brain dump,"*** it's a method to understand, process, and release lingering thoughts that have built up throughout the day. Doing so will help to reduce stress and pave the way for a more peaceful night.

Thoughts/feelings

Use this space to let go of everything on your mind and write down your thoughts and feelings (from fleeting thoughts to deepest emotions). Writing them down without feeling "judged" helps you understand your feelings and prevents nighttime overthinking as you drift off to sleep.

Highlights and Today's Wins

What made you smile, feel proud, or brought you a sense of accomplishment today? Celebrate even the smallest wins and what you are especially thankful for here.

2
WEEK

Evening Reflections

Declutter Your Mind

Steps to Prepare For Tomorrow

Consider today's challenges. Which moments or areas is there room for growth or change? What steps can you take for a "better" tomorrow?

Rate Your Day

How would you describe your day on a scale of 1 to 10?
Use the emojis below as a guide, with 1 representing a difficult day and 10 symbolising an exceptional one...

1	2	3	4	5	6	7	8	9	10

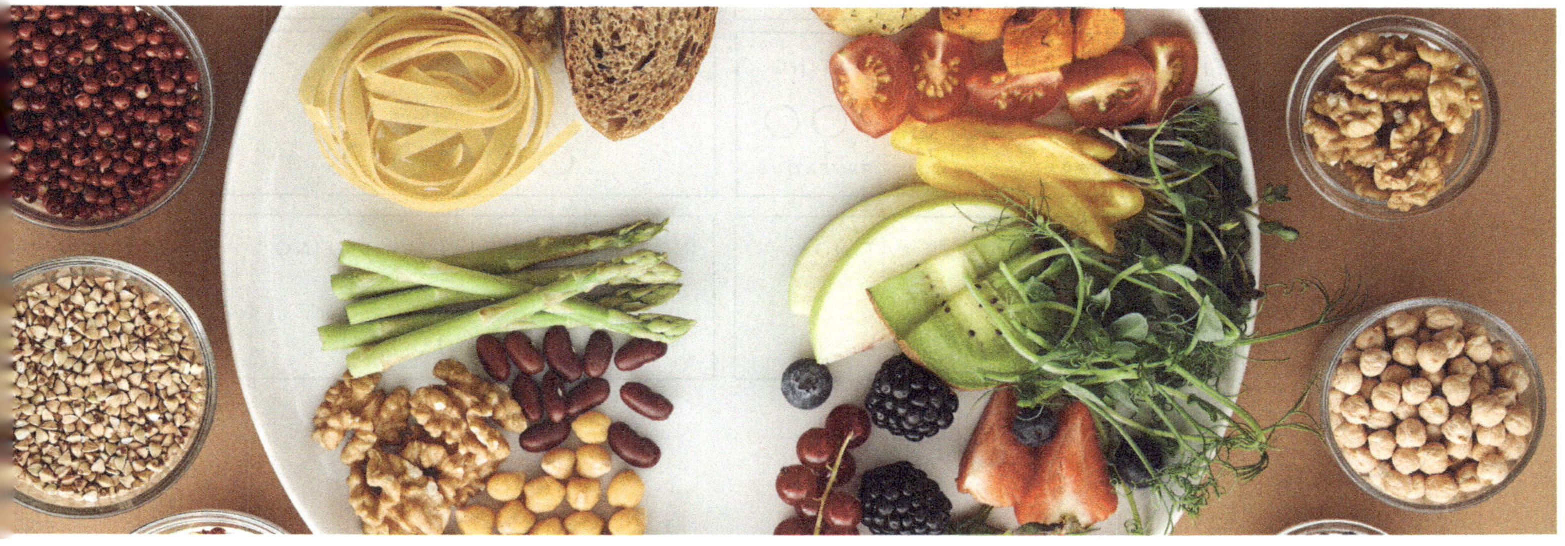

2
WEEK

Identifying Triggers

Day 4

Highlight any foods or drinks that seemed to worsen your symptoms during week one and monitor them closely during this week.

BREAKFAST

LUNCH

DINNER

SNACKS

DRINKS CONSUMED *(INCLUDING ALCOHOL)*

SUPPLEMENTS/MEDICATIONS TAKEN

HUNGER LEVELS BEFORE EATING

○ ○ ○ ○ ○ ○ ○ ○ ○ ○

1- NOT HUNGRY *10 - RAVENOUS*

MOOD BEFORE EATING

○ ○ ○ ○ ○

MOOD 1 HR AFTER EATING

○ ○ ○ ○ ○

MOOD 3 HRS AFTER EATING

○ ○ ○ ○ ○

BREAKFAST

LUNCH

DINNER

SNACKS

DRINKS CONSUMED *(INCLUDING ALCOHOL)*

SUPPLEMENTS/MEDICATIONS TAKEN

HUNGER LEVELS BEFORE EATING

○ ○ ○ ○ ○ ○ ○ ○ ○ ○

1- NOT HUNGRY *10 - RAVENOUS*

MOOD BEFORE EATING

○ ○ ○ ○ ○

MOOD 1 HR AFTER EATING

○ ○ ○ ○ ○

MOOD 3 HRS AFTER EATING

○ ○ ○ ○ ○

2 WEEK

Identifying Triggers

Day 4

Highlight any foods or drinks that seemed to worsen your symptoms during week one and monitor them closely during this week.

BREAKFAST

LUNCH

DINNER

SNACKS

DRINKS CONSUMED *(INCLUDING ALCOHOL)*

SUPPLEMENTS/MEDICATIONS TAKEN

HUNGER LEVELS BEFORE EATING

○ ○ ○ ○ ○ ○ ○ ○ ○ ○

1- NOT HUNGRY *10 - RAVENOUS*

MOOD BEFORE EATING

○ ○ ○ ○ ○

MOOD 1 HR AFTER EATING

○ ○ ○ ○ ○

MOOD 3 HRS AFTER EATING

○ ○ ○ ○ ○

BREAKFAST

LUNCH

DINNER

SNACKS

DRINKS CONSUMED *(INCLUDING ALCOHOL)*

SUPPLEMENTS/MEDICATIONS TAKEN

HUNGER LEVELS BEFORE EATING

○ ○ ○ ○ ○ ○ ○ ○ ○ ○

1- NOT HUNGRY *10 - RAVENOUS*

MOOD BEFORE EATING

○ ○ ○ ○ ○

MOOD 1 HR AFTER EATING

○ ○ ○ ○ ○

MOOD 3 HRS AFTER EATING

○ ○ ○ ○ ○

2 WEEK

Identifying Triggers

Highlight any foods or drinks that seemed to worsen your symptoms during week one and monitor them closely during this week.

Observations

____

____

____

____

____

____

- ☐ Bloating
- ☐ Energy Spike
- ☐ Irritability
- ☐ Headache
- ☐ Skin Reaction
- ☐ Nausea
- ☐ Vomiting
- ☐ Constipation
- ☐ Diarrhea
- ☐ Gas
- ☐ Other (*space for them to explain*)

____

Perimenopausal/Menopausal Symptoms

Symptoms Experienced

- ☐ Hot Flashes
- ☐ Sweating
- ☐ Night Sweats
- ☐ Anxiety
- ☐ Bloating
- ☐ Fatigue
- ☐ Gas
- ☐ Brain Fog
- ☐ Poor Concentration
- ☐ Mood Swings
- ☐ Cravings
- ☐ Sleep Disturbances
- ☐ Vaginal Dryness
- ☐ Headache
- ☐ Other (please explain)

____

☐ Mild ☐ Moderate ☐ Severe

Duration of Symptoms

____

____

____

____

____

____

____

☐ 5 Mins ☐ 15 Mins ☐ 1 Hour

New Symptoms:
Please explain

____

____

____

____

Observations:
Please explain

____

____

____

____

2
WEEK

Identifying Triggers

Breastfeeding / Pumping Information

TIME	FEEDING / PUMPING		SLEEP OR ACTIVITY	BABY TOILETING	
	DURATION (Feeding)	AMOUNT (Bottle/ Pump)		PEE	POOP

Feelings & Observations

2
WEEK

Evening Reflections

Declutter Your Mind

As the day ends, take a moment to ***reflect on your day,*** and use this space to ***declutter your mind.*** Jot down your thoughts, feelings, and any moments that stood out. ***Often referred to as a "brain dump,"*** it's a method to understand, process, and release lingering thoughts that have built up throughout the day. Doing so will help to reduce stress and pave the way for a more peaceful night.

Thoughts/feelings

Use this space to let go of everything on your mind and write down your thoughts and feelings (from fleeting thoughts to deepest emotions). Writing them down without feeling "judged" helps you understand your feelings and prevents nighttime overthinking as you drift off to sleep.

Highlights and Today's Wins

What made you smile, feel proud, or brought you a sense of accomplishment today? Celebrate even the smallest wins and what you are especially thankful for here.

2 WEEK

Evening Reflections

Declutter Your Mind

Steps to Prepare For Tomorrow

Consider today's challenges. Which moments or areas is there room for growth or change? What steps can you take for a "better" tomorrow?

Rate Your Day

How would you describe your day on a scale of 1 to 10?
Use the emojis below as a guide, with 1 representing a difficult day and 10 symbolising an exceptional one...

1	2	3	4	5	6	7	8	9	10

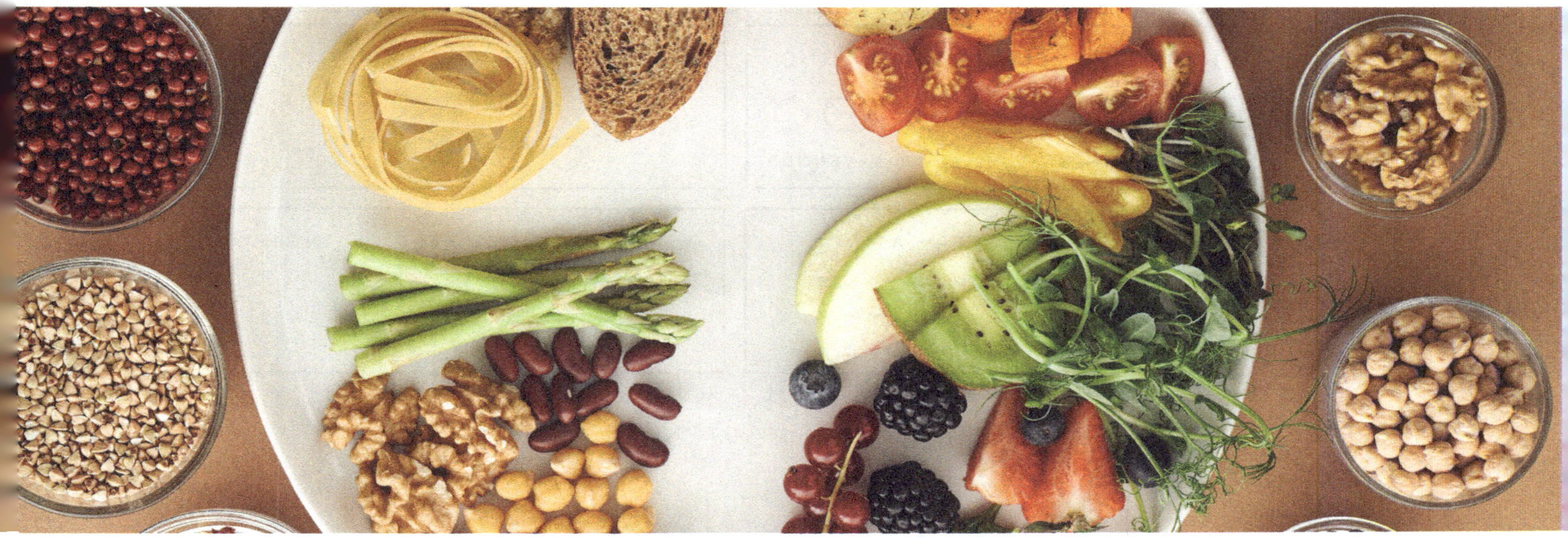

2 WEEK

Identifying Triggers

Day 5

Highlight any foods or drinks that seemed to worsen your symptoms during week one and monitor them closely during this week.

BREAKFAST

LUNCH

DINNER

SNACKS

DRINKS CONSUMED *(INCLUDING ALCOHOL)*

SUPPLEMENTS/MEDICATIONS TAKEN

HUNGER LEVELS BEFORE EATING

○ ○ ○ ○ ○ ○ ○ ○ ○ ○

1- NOT HUNGRY *10 - RAVENOUS*

MOOD BEFORE EATING

○ ○ ○ ○ ○

MOOD 1 HR AFTER EATING

○ ○ ○ ○ ○

MOOD 3 HRS AFTER EATING

○ ○ ○ ○ ○

BREAKFAST

LUNCH

DINNER

SNACKS

DRINKS CONSUMED *(INCLUDING ALCOHOL)*

SUPPLEMENTS/MEDICATIONS TAKEN

HUNGER LEVELS BEFORE EATING

○ ○ ○ ○ ○ ○ ○ ○ ○ ○

1- NOT HUNGRY *10 - RAVENOUS*

MOOD BEFORE EATING

○ ○ ○ ○ ○

MOOD 1 HR AFTER EATING

○ ○ ○ ○ ○

MOOD 3 HRS AFTER EATING

○ ○ ○ ○ ○

2
WEEK

Identifying Triggers

Day 5

Highlight any foods or drinks that seemed to worsen your symptoms during week one and monitor them closely during this week.

BREAKFAST

LUNCH

DINNER

SNACKS

DRINKS CONSUMED *(INCLUDING ALCOHOL)*

SUPPLEMENTS/MEDICATIONS TAKEN

HUNGER LEVELS BEFORE EATING

○ ○ ○ ○ ○ ○ ○ ○ ○ ○

1- NOT HUNGRY *10 - RAVENOUS*

MOOD BEFORE EATING

○ ○ ○ ○ ○

MOOD 1 HR AFTER EATING

○ ○ ○ ○ ○

MOOD 3 HRS AFTER EATING

○ ○ ○ ○ ○

BREAKFAST

LUNCH

DINNER

SNACKS

DRINKS CONSUMED *(INCLUDING ALCOHOL)*

SUPPLEMENTS/MEDICATIONS TAKEN

HUNGER LEVELS BEFORE EATING

○ ○ ○ ○ ○ ○ ○ ○ ○ ○

1- NOT HUNGRY *10 - RAVENOUS*

MOOD BEFORE EATING

○ ○ ○ ○ ○

MOOD 1 HR AFTER EATING

○ ○ ○ ○ ○

MOOD 3 HRS AFTER EATING

○ ○ ○ ○ ○

2 WEEK

Identifying Triggers

Highlight any foods or drinks that seemed to worsen your symptoms during week one and monitor them closely during this week.

Observations

____

____

____

____

____

____

- [ ] Bloating
- [ ] Energy Spike
- [ ] Irritability
- [ ] Headache
- [ ] Skin Reaction
- [ ] Nausea
- [ ] Vomiting
- [ ] Constipation
- [ ] Diarrhea
- [ ] Gas
- [ ] Other *(space for them to explain)*

____

Perimenopausal/Menopausal Symptoms

Symptoms Experienced

- [ ] Hot Flashes
- [ ] Sweating
- [ ] Night Sweats
- [ ] Anxiety
- [ ] Bloating
- [ ] Fatigue
- [ ] Gas
- [ ] Brain Fog
- [ ] Poor Concentration
- [ ] Mood Swings
- [ ] Cravings
- [ ] Sleep Disturbances
- [ ] Vaginal Dryness
- [ ] Headache
- [ ] Other (please explain)

____

- [ ] Mild
- [ ] Moderate
- [ ] Severe

Duration of Symptoms

____

____

____

____

____

____

____

- [ ] 5 Mins
- [ ] 15 Mins
- [ ] 1 Hour

New Symptoms:

Please explain

____

____

____

____

Observations:

Please explain

____

____

____

____

2 WEEK Identifying Triggers

Breastfeeding / Pumping Information

TIME	FEEDING / PUMPING		SLEEP OR ACTIVITY	BABY TOILETING	
	DURATION (Feeding)	AMOUNT (Bottle/ Pump)		PEE	POOP

Feelings & Observations

2
WEEK

Evening Reflections

Declutter Your Mind

As the day ends, take a moment to ***reflect on your day,*** and use this space to ***declutter your mind.*** Jot down your thoughts, feelings, and any moments that stood out. ***Often referred to as a "brain dump,"*** it's a method to understand, process, and release lingering thoughts that have built up throughout the day. Doing so will help to reduce stress and pave the way for a more peaceful night.

Thoughts/feelings

Use this space to let go of everything on your mind and write down your thoughts and feelings (from fleeting thoughts to deepest emotions). Writing them down without feeling "judged" helps you understand your feelings and prevents nighttime overthinking as you drift off to sleep.

Highlights and Today's Wins

What made you smile, feel proud, or brought you a sense of accomplishment today? Celebrate even the smallest wins and what you are especially thankful for here.

WEEK 2

Evening Reflections

Declutter Your Mind

Steps to Prepare For Tomorrow

Consider today's challenges. Which moments or areas is there room for growth or change? What steps can you take for a "better" tomorrow?

Rate Your Day

How would you describe your day on a scale of 1 to 10?
Use the emojis below as a guide, with 1 representing a difficult day and 10 symbolising an exceptional one...

1	2	3	4	5	6	7	8	9	10

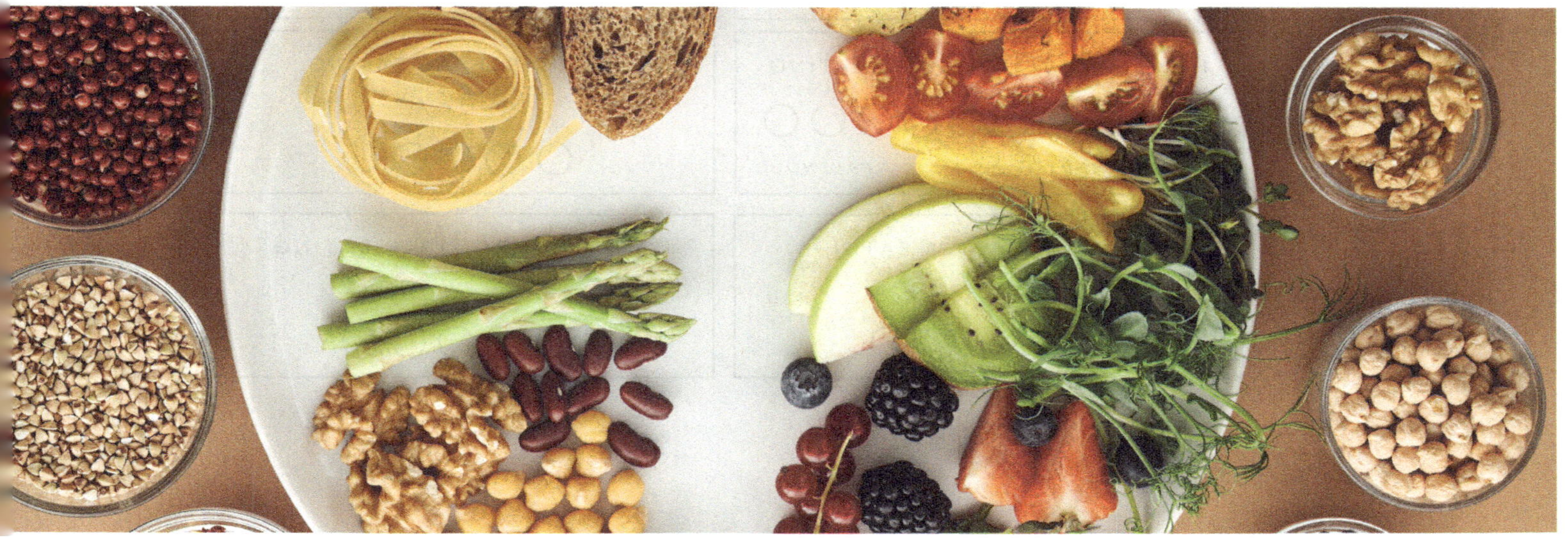

2
WEEK

Identifying Triggers

Day 6

Highlight any foods or drinks that seemed to worsen your symptoms during week one and monitor them closely during this week.

BREAKFAST

LUNCH

DINNER

SNACKS

DRINKS CONSUMED *(INCLUDING ALCOHOL)*

SUPPLEMENTS/MEDICATIONS TAKEN

HUNGER LEVELS BEFORE EATING

○ ○ ○ ○ ○ ○ ○ ○ ○ ○

1- NOT HUNGRY *10 - RAVENOUS*

MOOD BEFORE EATING

○ ○ ○ ○ ○

MOOD 1 HR AFTER EATING

○ ○ ○ ○ ○

MOOD 3 HRS AFTER EATING

○ ○ ○ ○ ○

BREAKFAST

LUNCH

DINNER

SNACKS

DRINKS CONSUMED *(INCLUDING ALCOHOL)*

SUPPLEMENTS/MEDICATIONS TAKEN

HUNGER LEVELS BEFORE EATING

○ ○ ○ ○ ○ ○ ○ ○ ○ ○

1- NOT HUNGRY *10 - RAVENOUS*

MOOD BEFORE EATING

○ ○ ○ ○ ○

MOOD 1 HR AFTER EATING

○ ○ ○ ○ ○

MOOD 3 HRS AFTER EATING

○ ○ ○ ○ ○

2
WEEK

Identifying Triggers

Day 6

Highlight any foods or drinks that seemed to worsen your symptoms during week one and monitor them closely during this week.

BREAKFAST

LUNCH

DINNER

SNACKS

DRINKS CONSUMED *(INCLUDING ALCOHOL)*

SUPPLEMENTS/MEDICATIONS TAKEN

HUNGER LEVELS BEFORE EATING

○ ○ ○ ○ ○ ○ ○ ○ ○ ○

1- NOT HUNGRY *10 - RAVENOUS*

MOOD BEFORE EATING

○ ○ ○ ○ ○

MOOD 1 HR AFTER EATING

○ ○ ○ ○ ○

MOOD 3 HRS AFTER EATING

○ ○ ○ ○ ○

BREAKFAST

LUNCH

DINNER

SNACKS

DRINKS CONSUMED *(INCLUDING ALCOHOL)*

SUPPLEMENTS/MEDICATIONS TAKEN

HUNGER LEVELS BEFORE EATING

○ ○ ○ ○ ○ ○ ○ ○ ○ ○

1- NOT HUNGRY *10 - RAVENOUS*

MOOD BEFORE EATING

○ ○ ○ ○ ○

MOOD 1 HR AFTER EATING

○ ○ ○ ○ ○

MOOD 3 HRS AFTER EATING

○ ○ ○ ○ ○

2
WEEK

Identifying Triggers

Highlight any foods or drinks that seemed to worsen your symptoms during week one and monitor them closely during this week.

Observations

- [ ] Bloating
- [ ] Energy Spike
- [ ] Irritability
- [ ] Headache
- [ ] Skin Reaction
- [ ] Nausea
- [ ] Vomiting
- [ ] Constipation
- [ ] Diarrhea
- [ ] Gas
- [ ] Other *(space for them to explain)*

Perimenopausal/Menopausal Symptoms

Symptoms Experienced

- [ ] Hot Flashes
- [ ] Sweating
- [ ] Night Sweats
- [ ] Anxiety
- [ ] Bloating
- [ ] Fatigue
- [ ] Gas
- [ ] Brain Fog
- [ ] Poor Concentration
- [ ] Mood Swings
- [ ] Cravings
- [ ] Sleep Disturbances
- [ ] Vaginal Dryness
- [ ] Headache
- [ ] Other (please explain)

- [ ] Mild
- [ ] Moderate
- [ ] Severe

Duration of Symptoms

- [ ] 5 Mins
- [ ] 15 Mins
- [ ] 1 Hour

New Symptoms:

Please explain

Observations:

Please explain

2
WEEK

Identifying Triggers

Breastfeeding / Pumping Information

TIME	FEEDING / PUMPING		SLEEP OR ACTIVITY	BABY TOILETING	
	DURATION (Feeding)	AMOUNT (Bottle/ Pump)		PEE	POOP

Feelings & Observations

2
WEEK

Evening Reflections

Declutter Your Mind

As the day ends, take a moment to ***reflect on your day,*** and use this space to ***declutter your mind.*** Jot down your thoughts, feelings, and any moments that stood out. ***Often referred to as a "brain dump,"*** it's a method to understand, process, and release lingering thoughts that have built up throughout the day. Doing so will help to reduce stress and pave the way for a more peaceful night.

Thoughts/feelings

Use this space to let go of everything on your mind and write down your thoughts and feelings (from fleeting thoughts to deepest emotions). Writing them down without feeling "judged" helps you understand your feelings and prevents nighttime overthinking as you drift off to sleep.

Highlights and Today's Wins

What made you smile, feel proud, or brought you a sense of accomplishment today? Celebrate even the smallest wins and what you are especially thankful for here.

2
WEEK

Evening Reflections

Declutter Your Mind

Steps to Prepare For Tomorrow

Consider today's challenges. Which moments or areas is there room for growth or change? What steps can you take for a "better" tomorrow?

Rate Your Day

How would you describe your day on a scale of 1 to 10?
Use the emojis below as a guide, with 1 representing a difficult day and 10 symbolising an exceptional one...

1	2	3	4	5	6	7	8	9	10

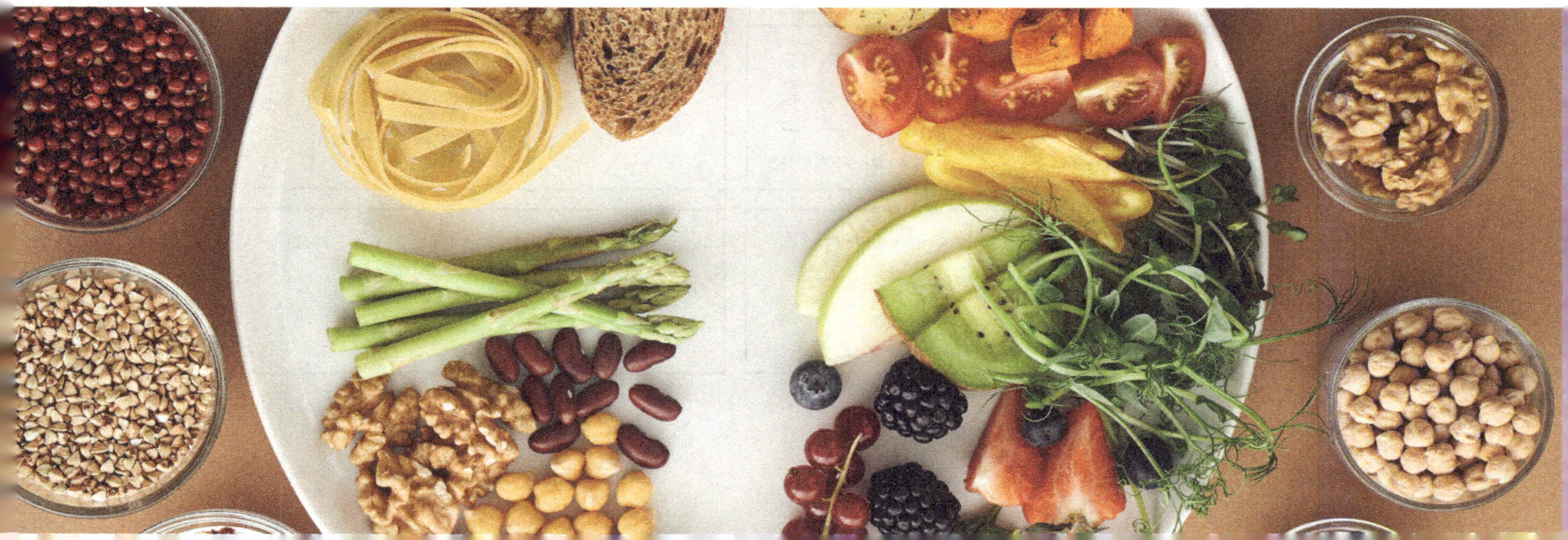

2 WEEK

Identifying Triggers

Day 7

Highlight any foods or drinks that seemed to worsen your symptoms during week one and monitor them closely during this week.

BREAKFAST

LUNCH

DINNER

SNACKS

DRINKS CONSUMED *(INCLUDING ALCOHOL)*

SUPPLEMENTS/MEDICATIONS TAKEN

HUNGER LEVELS BEFORE EATING

○○○○○○○○○○

1- NOT HUNGRY *10 - RAVENOUS*

MOOD BEFORE EATING

○○○○○

MOOD 1 HR AFTER EATING

○○○○○

MOOD 3 HRS AFTER EATING

○○○○○

BREAKFAST

LUNCH

DINNER

SNACKS

DRINKS CONSUMED *(INCLUDING ALCOHOL)*

SUPPLEMENTS/MEDICATIONS TAKEN

HUNGER LEVELS BEFORE EATING

○○○○○○○○○○

1- NOT HUNGRY *10 - RAVENOUS*

MOOD BEFORE EATING

○○○○○

MOOD 1 HR AFTER EATING

○○○○○

MOOD 3 HRS AFTER EATING

○○○○○

Identifying Triggers

Day 7

Highlight any foods or drinks that seemed to worsen your symptoms during week one and monitor them closely during this week.

BREAKFAST

LUNCH

DINNER

SNACKS

DRINKS CONSUMED *(INCLUDING ALCOHOL)*

SUPPLEMENTS/MEDICATIONS TAKEN

HUNGER LEVELS BEFORE EATING

1- NOT HUNGRY *10 - RAVENOUS*

MOOD BEFORE EATING

MOOD 1 HR AFTER EATING

MOOD 3 HRS AFTER EATING

BREAKFAST

LUNCH

DINNER

SNACKS

DRINKS CONSUMED *(INCLUDING ALCOHOL)*

SUPPLEMENTS/MEDICATIONS TAKEN

HUNGER LEVELS BEFORE EATING

1- NOT HUNGRY *10 - RAVENOUS*

MOOD BEFORE EATING

MOOD 1 HR AFTER EATING

MOOD 3 HRS AFTER EATING

2 WEEK

Identifying Triggers

Highlight any foods or drinks that seemed to worsen your symptoms during week one and monitor them closely during this week.

Observations

____
____
____
____
____
____

- ☐ Bloating
- ☐ Energy Spike
- ☐ Irritability
- ☐ Headache
- ☐ Skin Reaction
- ☐ Nausea
- ☐ Vomiting
- ☐ Constipation
- ☐ Diarrhea
- ☐ Gas
- ☐ Other *(space for them to explain)* ______________________________

Perimenopausal/Menopausal Symptoms

Symptoms Experienced

- ☐ Hot Flashes
- ☐ Sweating
- ☐ Night Sweats
- ☐ Anxiety
- ☐ Bloating
- ☐ Fatigue
- ☐ Gas
- ☐ Brain Fog
- ☐ Poor Concentration
- ☐ Mood Swings
- ☐ Cravings
- ☐ Sleep Disturbances
- ☐ Vaginal Dryness
- ☐ Headache
- ☐ Other (please explain) ______________________________

☐ Mild ☐ Moderate ☐ Severe

Duration of Symptoms

____
____
____
____
____
____
____

☐ 5 Mins ☐ 15 Mins ☐ 1 Hour

New Symptoms:

Please explain

____
____
____
____

Observations:

Please explain

____
____
____
____

2 WEEK

Identifying Triggers

Breastfeeding / Pumping Information

TIME	FEEDING / PUMPING		SLEEP OR ACTIVITY	BABY TOILETING	
	DURATION (Feeding)	AMOUNT (Bottle/ Pump)		PEE	POOP

Feelings & Observations

2
WEEK

Evening Reflections

Declutter Your Mind

As the day ends, take a moment to ***reflect on your day,*** and use this space to ***declutter your mind.*** Jot down your thoughts, feelings, and any moments that stood out. ***Often referred to as a "brain dump,"*** it's a method to understand, process, and release lingering thoughts that have built up throughout the day. Doing so will help to reduce stress and pave the way for a more peaceful night.

Thoughts/feelings

Use this space to let go of everything on your mind and write down your thoughts and feelings (from fleeting thoughts to deepest emotions). Writing them down without feeling "judged" helps you understand your feelings and prevents nighttime overthinking as you drift off to sleep.

Highlights and Today's Wins

What made you smile, feel proud, or brought you a sense of accomplishment today? Celebrate even the smallest wins and what you are especially thankful for here.

Evening Reflections

Declutter Your Mind

Steps to Prepare For Tomorrow

Consider today's challenges. Which moments or areas is there room for growth or change? What steps can you take for a "better" tomorrow?

Rate Your Day

How would you describe your day on a scale of 1 to 10?
Use the emojis below as a guide, with 1 representing a difficult day and 10 symbolising an exceptional one...

1	2	3	4	5	6	7	8	9	10

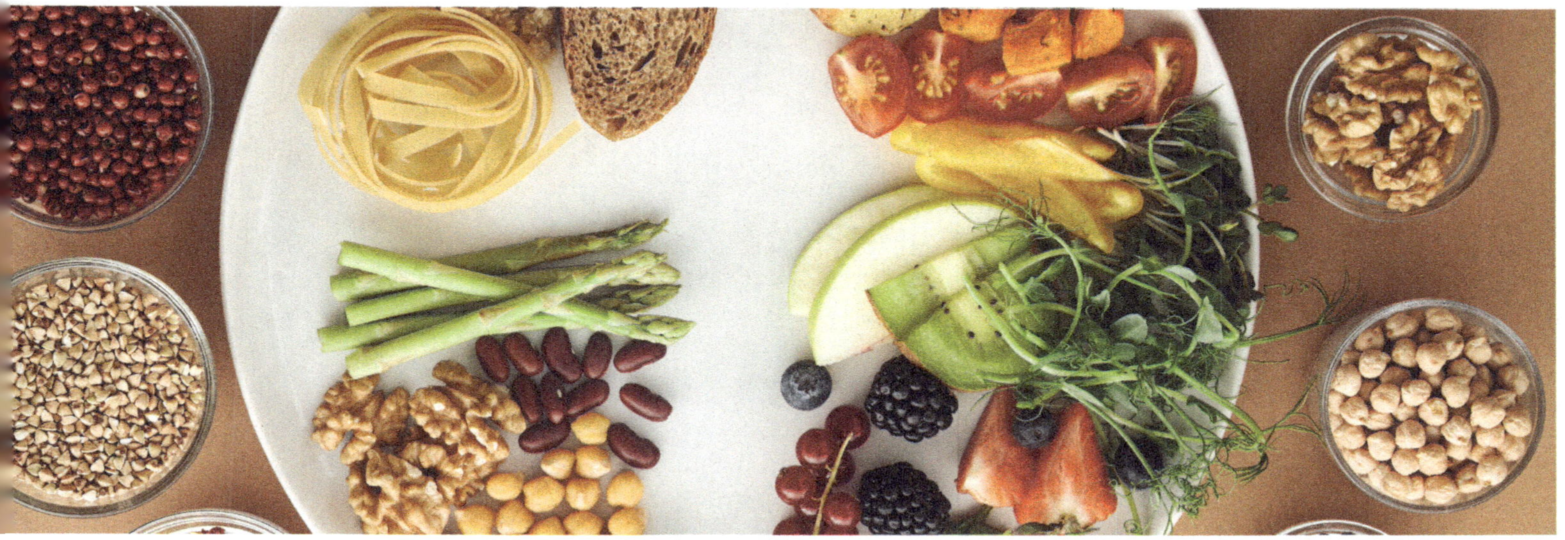

3 WEEK

Food & Drink Removal

Day 1

Remove specific foods and drinks identified in Week 2 from your diet and observe any changes in your symptoms.

BREAKFAST

LUNCH

DINNER

SNACKS

DRINKS CONSUMED *(INCLUDING ALCOHOL)*

SUPPLEMENTS/MEDICATIONS TAKEN

HUNGER LEVELS BEFORE EATING

○ ○ ○ ○ ○ ○ ○ ○ ○ ○

1- NOT HUNGRY *10 - RAVENOUS*

MOOD BEFORE EATING

○ ○ ○ ○ ○

MOOD 1 HR AFTER EATING

○ ○ ○ ○ ○

MOOD 3 HRS AFTER EATING

○ ○ ○ ○ ○

BREAKFAST

LUNCH

DINNER

SNACKS

DRINKS CONSUMED *(INCLUDING ALCOHOL)*

SUPPLEMENTS/MEDICATIONS TAKEN

HUNGER LEVELS BEFORE EATING

○ ○ ○ ○ ○ ○ ○ ○ ○ ○

1- NOT HUNGRY *10 - RAVENOUS*

MOOD BEFORE EATING

○ ○ ○ ○ ○

MOOD 1 HR AFTER EATING

○ ○ ○ ○ ○

MOOD 3 HRS AFTER EATING

○ ○ ○ ○ ○

3 WEEK

Food & Drink Removal

Day 1

Remove specific foods and drinks identified in Week 2 from your diet and observe any changes in your symptoms.

BREAKFAST

LUNCH

DINNER

SNACKS

DRINKS CONSUMED *(INCLUDING ALCOHOL)*

SUPPLEMENTS/MEDICATIONS TAKEN

HUNGER LEVELS BEFORE EATING

○ ○ ○ ○ ○ ○ ○ ○ ○ ○

1- NOT HUNGRY *10 - RAVENOUS*

MOOD BEFORE EATING

○ ○ ○ ○ ○

MOOD 1 HR AFTER EATING

○ ○ ○ ○ ○

MOOD 3 HRS AFTER EATING

○ ○ ○ ○ ○

BREAKFAST

LUNCH

DINNER

SNACKS

DRINKS CONSUMED *(INCLUDING ALCOHOL)*

SUPPLEMENTS/MEDICATIONS TAKEN

HUNGER LEVELS BEFORE EATING

○ ○ ○ ○ ○ ○ ○ ○ ○ ○

1- NOT HUNGRY *10 - RAVENOUS*

MOOD BEFORE EATING

○ ○ ○ ○ ○

MOOD 1 HR AFTER EATING

○ ○ ○ ○ ○

MOOD 3 HRS AFTER EATING

○ ○ ○ ○ ○

3
WEEK

Food & Drink Removal

Remove specific foods and drinks identified in Week 2 from your diet and observe any changes in your symptoms.

Observations

- [ ] Bloating
- [ ] Energy Spike
- [ ] Irritability
- [ ] Headache
- [ ] Skin Reaction
- [ ] Nausea
- [ ] Vomiting
- [ ] Constipation
- [ ] Diarrhea
- [ ] Gas
- [ ] Other *(space for them to explain)*

Perimenopausal/Menopausal Symptoms

Symptoms Experienced

- [ ] Hot Flashes
- [ ] Sweating
- [ ] Night Sweats
- [ ] Anxiety
- [ ] Bloating
- [ ] Fatigue
- [ ] Gas
- [ ] Brain Fog
- [ ] Poor Concentration
- [ ] Mood Swings
- [ ] Cravings
- [ ] Sleep Disturbances
- [ ] Vaginal Dryness
- [ ] Headache
- [ ] Other (please explain)

- [ ] Mild
- [ ] Moderate
- [ ] Severe

Duration of Symptoms

- [ ] 5 Mins
- [ ] 15 Mins
- [ ] 1 Hour

New Symptoms:

Please explain

Observations:

Please explain

3
WEEK

Food & Drink Removal

Remove specific foods and drinks identified in Week 2 from your diet and observe any changes in your symptoms.

Physical Activity

Type of Activity:

Duration:

Intensity:

☐ Low ☐ Moderate ☐ High

Sleep

Quality of Sleep:

☐ Excellent ☐ Poor
☐ Good ☐ Very Poor
☐ Fair

Hours Slept:

____

____

____

Support System:

Stress Management Techniques:

Water Intake Tracker:

💧 💧 💧 💧 💧 💧 💧 💧

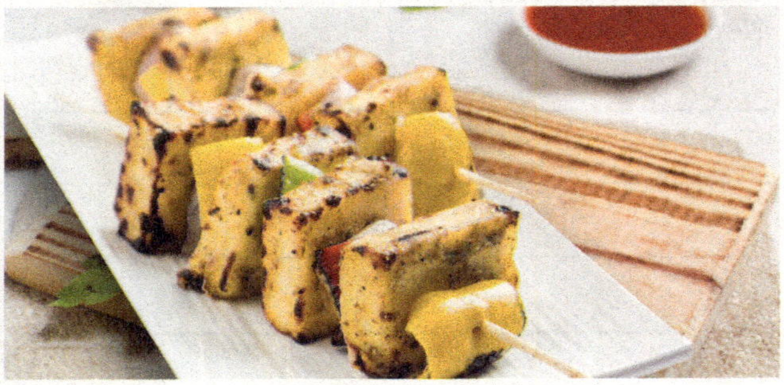

Overall Observations for the Day:

3
WEEK

Food & Drink Removal

Breastfeeding / Pumping Information

TIME	FEEDING / PUMPING		SLEEP OR ACTIVITY	BABY TOILETING	
	DURATION (Feeding)	AMOUNT (Bottle/ Pump)		PEE	POOP

Feelings & Observations

3 WEEK

Evening Reflections

Declutter Your Mind

As the day ends, take a moment to ***reflect on your day,*** and use this space to ***declutter your mind.*** Jot down your thoughts, feelings, and any moments that stood out. ***Often referred to as a "brain dump,"*** it's a method to understand, process, and release lingering thoughts that have built up throughout the day. Doing so will help to reduce stress and pave the way for a more peaceful night.

Thoughts/feelings

Use this space to let go of everything on your mind and write down your thoughts and feelings (from fleeting thoughts to deepest emotions). Writing them down without feeling "judged" helps you understand your feelings and prevents nighttime overthinking as you drift off to sleep.

Highlights and Today's Wins

What made you smile, feel proud, or brought you a sense of accomplishment today? Celebrate even the smallest wins and what you are especially thankful for here.

3 WEEK

Evening Reflections

Declutter Your Mind

Steps to Prepare For Tomorrow

Consider today's challenges. Which moments or areas is there room for growth or change? What steps can you take for a "better" tomorrow?

____

____

____

____

____

____

____

Rate Your Day

How would you describe your day on a scale of 1 to 10?
Use the emojis below as a guide, with 1 representing a difficult day and 10 symbolising an exceptional one...

1	2	3	4	5	6	7	8	9	10

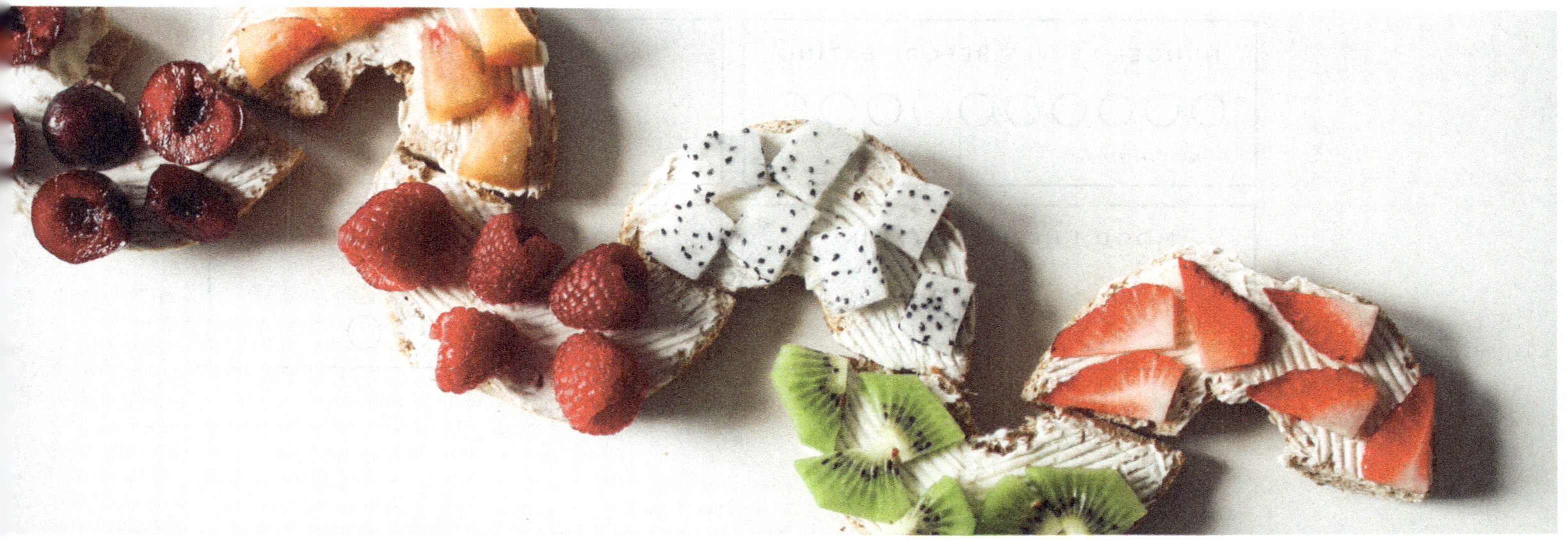

3
WEEK

Food & Drink Removal

Day 2

Remove specific foods and drinks identified in Week 2 from your diet and observe any changes in your symptoms.

BREAKFAST

LUNCH

DINNER

SNACKS

DRINKS CONSUMED *(INCLUDING ALCOHOL)*

SUPPLEMENTS/MEDICATIONS TAKEN

HUNGER LEVELS BEFORE EATING

○ ○ ○ ○ ○ ○ ○ ○ ○ ○

1- NOT HUNGRY *10 - RAVENOUS*

MOOD BEFORE EATING

○ ○ ○ ○ ○

MOOD 1 HR AFTER EATING

○ ○ ○ ○ ○

MOOD 3 HRS AFTER EATING

○ ○ ○ ○ ○

BREAKFAST

LUNCH

DINNER

SNACKS

DRINKS CONSUMED *(INCLUDING ALCOHOL)*

SUPPLEMENTS/MEDICATIONS TAKEN

HUNGER LEVELS BEFORE EATING

○ ○ ○ ○ ○ ○ ○ ○ ○ ○

1- NOT HUNGRY *10 - RAVENOUS*

MOOD BEFORE EATING

○ ○ ○ ○ ○

MOOD 1 HR AFTER EATING

○ ○ ○ ○ ○

MOOD 3 HRS AFTER EATING

○ ○ ○ ○ ○

3 WEEK

Food & Drink Removal

Day 2

Remove specific foods and drinks identified in Week 2 from your diet and observe any changes in your symptoms.

BREAKFAST

LUNCH

DINNER

SNACKS

DRINKS CONSUMED *(INCLUDING ALCOHOL)*

SUPPLEMENTS/MEDICATIONS TAKEN

HUNGER LEVELS BEFORE EATING

○ ○ ○ ○ ○ ○ ○ ○ ○ ○

1- NOT HUNGRY *10 - RAVENOUS*

MOOD BEFORE EATING

○ ○ ○ ○ ○

MOOD 1 HR AFTER EATING

○ ○ ○ ○ ○

MOOD 3 HRS AFTER EATING

○ ○ ○ ○ ○

BREAKFAST

LUNCH

DINNER

SNACKS

DRINKS CONSUMED *(INCLUDING ALCOHOL)*

SUPPLEMENTS/MEDICATIONS TAKEN

HUNGER LEVELS BEFORE EATING

○ ○ ○ ○ ○ ○ ○ ○ ○ ○

1- NOT HUNGRY *10 - RAVENOUS*

MOOD BEFORE EATING

○ ○ ○ ○ ○

MOOD 1 HR AFTER EATING

○ ○ ○ ○ ○

MOOD 3 HRS AFTER EATING

○ ○ ○ ○ ○

3
WEEK

Food & Drink Removal

Remove specific foods and drinks identified in Week 2 from your diet and observe any changes in your symptoms.

Physical Activity

Type of Activity:

Duration:

Intensity:

☐ Low ☐ Moderate ☐ High

Sleep

Quality of Sleep:

☐ Excellent
☐ Good
☐ Fair
☐ Poor
☐ Very Poor

Hours Slept:

Support System:

Stress Management Techniques:

Water Intake Tracker:

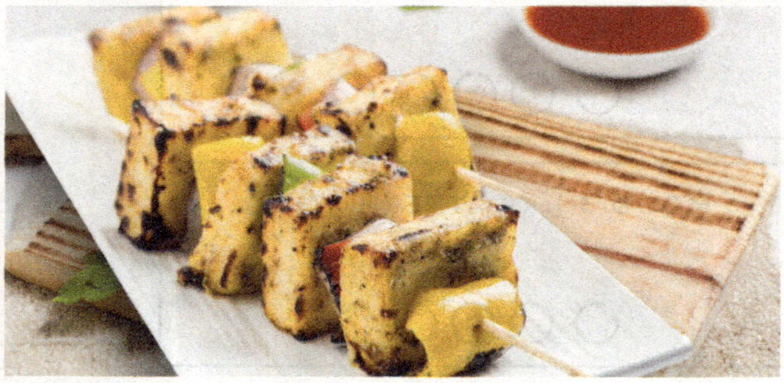

Overall Observations for the Day:

3
WEEK

Food & Drink Removal

Remove specific foods and drinks identified in Week 2 from your diet and observe any changes in your symptoms.

Observations

____
____
____
____
____
____

- ☐ Bloating
- ☐ Energy Spike
- ☐ Irritability
- ☐ Headache
- ☐ Skin Reaction
- ☐ Nausea
- ☐ Vomiting
- ☐ Constipation
- ☐ Diarrhea
- ☐ Gas
- ☐ Other *(space for them to explain)*

____

Perimenopausal/Menopausal Symptoms

Symptoms Experienced

- ☐ Hot Flashes
- ☐ Sweating
- ☐ Night Sweats
- ☐ Anxiety
- ☐ Bloating
- ☐ Fatigue
- ☐ Gas
- ☐ Brain Fog
- ☐ Poor Concentration
- ☐ Mood Swings
- ☐ Cravings
- ☐ Sleep Disturbances
- ☐ Vaginal Dryness
- ☐ Headache
- ☐ Other (please explain)

____

☐ Mild ☐ Moderate ☐ Severe

Duration of Symptoms

____
____
____
____
____
____
____

☐ 5 Mins ☐ 15 Mins ☐ 1 Hour

New Symptoms:

Please explain

____
____
____
____

Observations:

Please explain

____
____
____
____

3
WEEK

Food & Drink Removal

Remove specific foods and drinks identified in Week 2 from your diet and observe any changes in your symptoms.

Physical Activity

Type of Activity:

Duration:

Intensity:

☐ Low ☐ Moderate ☐ High

Sleep

Quality of Sleep:

☐ Excellent ☐ Poor
☐ Good ☐ Very Poor
☐ Fair

Hours Slept:

Support System:

Stress Management Techniques:

Water Intake Tracker:

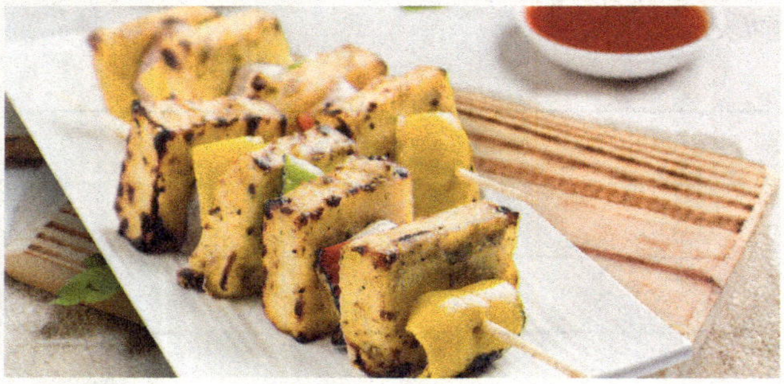

Overall Observations for the Day:

3 WEEK

Food & Drink Removal

Breastfeeding / Pumping Information

TIME	FEEDING / PUMPING		SLEEP OR ACTIVITY	BABY TOILETING	
	DURATION (Feeding)	AMOUNT (Bottle/ Pump)		PEE	POOP

Feelings & Observations

3
WEEK

Evening Reflections

Declutter Your Mind

As the day ends, take a moment to ***reflect on your day,*** and use this space to ***declutter your mind.*** Jot down your thoughts, feelings, and any moments that stood out. ***Often referred to as a "brain dump,"*** it's a method to understand, process, and release lingering thoughts that have built up throughout the day. Doing so will help to reduce stress and pave the way for a more peaceful night.

Thoughts/feelings

Use this space to let go of everything on your mind and write down your thoughts and feelings (from fleeting thoughts to deepest emotions). Writing them down without feeling "judged" helps you understand your feelings and prevents nighttime overthinking as you drift off to sleep.

Highlights and Today's Wins

What made you smile, feel proud, or brought you a sense of accomplishment today? Celebrate even the smallest wins and what you are especially thankful for here.

3
WEEK

Evening Reflections

Declutter Your Mind

Steps to Prepare For Tomorrow

Consider today's challenges. Which moments or areas is there room for growth or change? What steps can you take for a "better" tomorrow?

Rate Your Day

How would you describe your day on a scale of 1 to 10?
Use the emojis below as a guide, with 1 representing a difficult day and 10 symbolising an exceptional one...

1	2	3	4	5	6	7	8	9	10

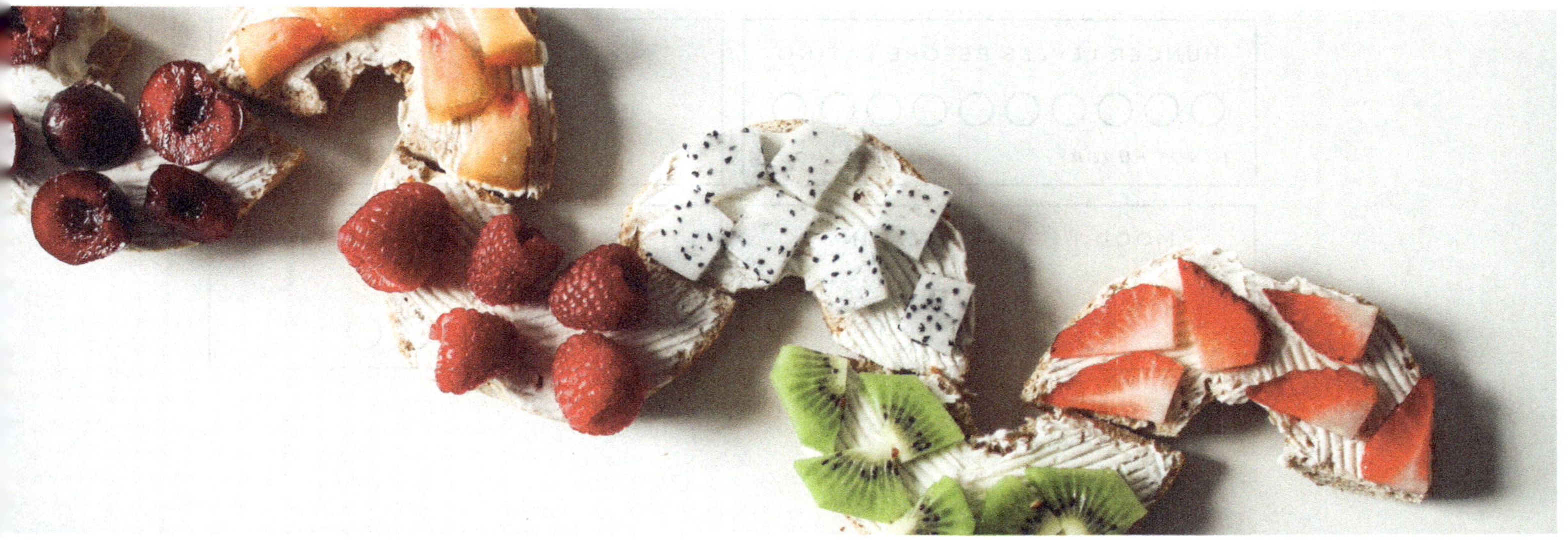

3 WEEK

Food & Drink Removal

Day 3

Remove specific foods and drinks identified in Week 2 from your diet and observe any changes in your symptoms.

BREAKFAST

LUNCH

DINNER

SNACKS

DRINKS CONSUMED *(INCLUDING ALCOHOL)*

SUPPLEMENTS/MEDICATIONS TAKEN

HUNGER LEVELS BEFORE EATING

○ ○ ○ ○ ○ ○ ○ ○ ○ ○

1- NOT HUNGRY *10 - RAVENOUS*

MOOD BEFORE EATING

○ ○ ○ ○ ○

MOOD 1 HR AFTER EATING

○ ○ ○ ○ ○

MOOD 3 HRS AFTER EATING

○ ○ ○ ○ ○

BREAKFAST

LUNCH

DINNER

SNACKS

DRINKS CONSUMED *(INCLUDING ALCOHOL)*

SUPPLEMENTS/MEDICATIONS TAKEN

HUNGER LEVELS BEFORE EATING

○ ○ ○ ○ ○ ○ ○ ○ ○ ○

1- NOT HUNGRY *10 - RAVENOUS*

MOOD BEFORE EATING

○ ○ ○ ○ ○

MOOD 1 HR AFTER EATING

○ ○ ○ ○ ○

MOOD 3 HRS AFTER EATING

○ ○ ○ ○ ○

3 WEEK

Food & Drink Removal

Day 3

Remove specific foods and drinks identified in Week 2 from your diet and observe any changes in your symptoms.

BREAKFAST

LUNCH

DINNER

SNACKS

DRINKS CONSUMED *(INCLUDING ALCOHOL)*

SUPPLEMENTS/MEDICATIONS TAKEN

HUNGER LEVELS BEFORE EATING

○ ○ ○ ○ ○ ○ ○ ○ ○ ○

1- NOT HUNGRY *10 - RAVENOUS*

MOOD BEFORE EATING

○ ○ ○ ○ ○

MOOD 1 HR AFTER EATING

○ ○ ○ ○ ○

MOOD 3 HRS AFTER EATING

○ ○ ○ ○ ○

BREAKFAST

LUNCH

DINNER

SNACKS

DRINKS CONSUMED *(INCLUDING ALCOHOL)*

SUPPLEMENTS/MEDICATIONS TAKEN

HUNGER LEVELS BEFORE EATING

○ ○ ○ ○ ○ ○ ○ ○ ○ ○

1- NOT HUNGRY *10 - RAVENOUS*

MOOD BEFORE EATING

○ ○ ○ ○ ○

MOOD 1 HR AFTER EATING

○ ○ ○ ○ ○

MOOD 3 HRS AFTER EATING

○ ○ ○ ○ ○

3
WEEK

Food & Drink Removal

Remove specific foods and drinks identified in Week 2 from your diet and observe any changes in your symptoms.

Day 4

Name: ______________________ **Date:** ______________

Meal Information

Meal Time:

Type of Meal:

☐ Breakfast ☐ Snack ☐ Lunch ☐ Dinner ☐ Late-night snack

Location:

☐ Home ☐ Work ☐ Restaurant ☐ On-the-go

Food & Drink Details

Food Item

Portion Size

Beverages

Feelings & Observations

Mood Before Eating

☐ Happy ☐ Relaxed ☐ Sad ☐ Stressed ☐ Neutral ☐ Hungry

☐ Not Hungry ☐ Other (please explain) ______________

Mood After Eating

☐ Satisfied ☐ Still Hungry ☐ Overfull ☐ Guilty ☐ Energised ☐ Sluggish

☐ Anxious ☐ Other (please explain) ______________

3
WEEK

Food & Drink Removal

Remove specific foods and drinks identified in Week 2 from your diet and observe any changes in your symptoms.

Observations

- [ ] Bloating
- [ ] Energy Spike
- [ ] Irritability
- [ ] Headache
- [ ] Skin Reaction
- [ ] Nausea
- [ ] Vomiting
- [ ] Constipation
- [ ] Diarrhea
- [ ] Gas
- [ ] Other *(space for them to explain)*

Perimenopausal/Menopausal Symptoms

Symptoms Experienced

- [ ] Hot Flashes
- [ ] Sweating
- [ ] Night Sweats
- [ ] Anxiety
- [ ] Bloating
- [ ] Fatigue
- [ ] Gas
- [ ] Brain Fog
- [ ] Poor Concentration
- [ ] Mood Swings
- [ ] Cravings
- [ ] Sleep Disturbances
- [ ] Vaginal Dryness
- [ ] Headache
- [ ] Other (please explain)

- [ ] Mild
- [ ] Moderate
- [ ] Severe

Duration of Symptoms

- [ ] 5 Mins
- [ ] 15 Mins
- [ ] 1 Hour

New Symptoms:

Please explain

Observations:

Please explain

3 WEEK

Food & Drink Removal

Remove specific foods and drinks identified in Week 2 from your diet and observe any changes in your symptoms.

Physical Activity

Type of Activity:

Duration:

Intensity:

☐ Low ☐ Moderate ☐ High

Sleep

Quality of Sleep:

☐ Excellent ☐ Poor
☐ Good ☐ Very Poor
☐ Fair

Hours Slept:

Support System:

Stress Management Techniques:

Water Intake Tracker:

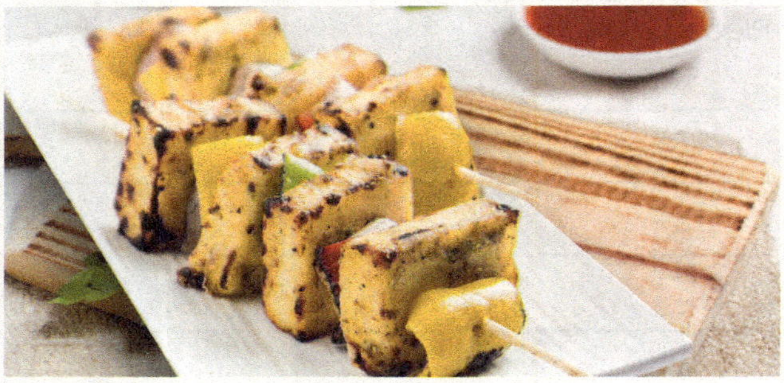

Overall Observations for the Day:

3 WEEK

Food & Drink Removal

Breastfeeding / Pumping Information

TIME	FEEDING / PUMPING		SLEEP OR ACTIVITY	BABY TOILETING	
	DURATION (Feeding)	AMOUNT (Bottle/ Pump)		PEE	POOP

Feelings & Observations

Evening Reflections

3
WEEK

Declutter Your Mind

As the day ends, take a moment to ***reflect on your day,*** and use this space to ***declutter your mind.*** Jot down your thoughts, feelings, and any moments that stood out. ***Often referred to as a "brain dump,"*** it's a method to understand, process, and release lingering thoughts that have built up throughout the day. Doing so will help to reduce stress and pave the way for a more peaceful night.

Thoughts/feelings

Use this space to let go of everything on your mind and write down your thoughts and feelings (from fleeting thoughts to deepest emotions). Writing them down without feeling "judged" helps you understand your feelings and prevents nighttime overthinking as you drift off to sleep.

Highlights and Today's Wins

What made you smile, feel proud, or brought you a sense of accomplishment today? Celebrate even the smallest wins and what you are especially thankful for here.

3
WEEK

Evening Reflections

Declutter Your Mind

Steps to Prepare For Tomorrow

Consider today's challenges. Which moments or areas is there room for growth or change? What steps can you take for a "better" tomorrow?

____

____

____

____

____

____

____

Rate Your Day

How would you describe your day on a scale of 1 to 10?
Use the emojis below as a guide, with 1 representing a difficult day and 10 symbolising an exceptional one...

1	2	3	4	5	6	7	8	9	10

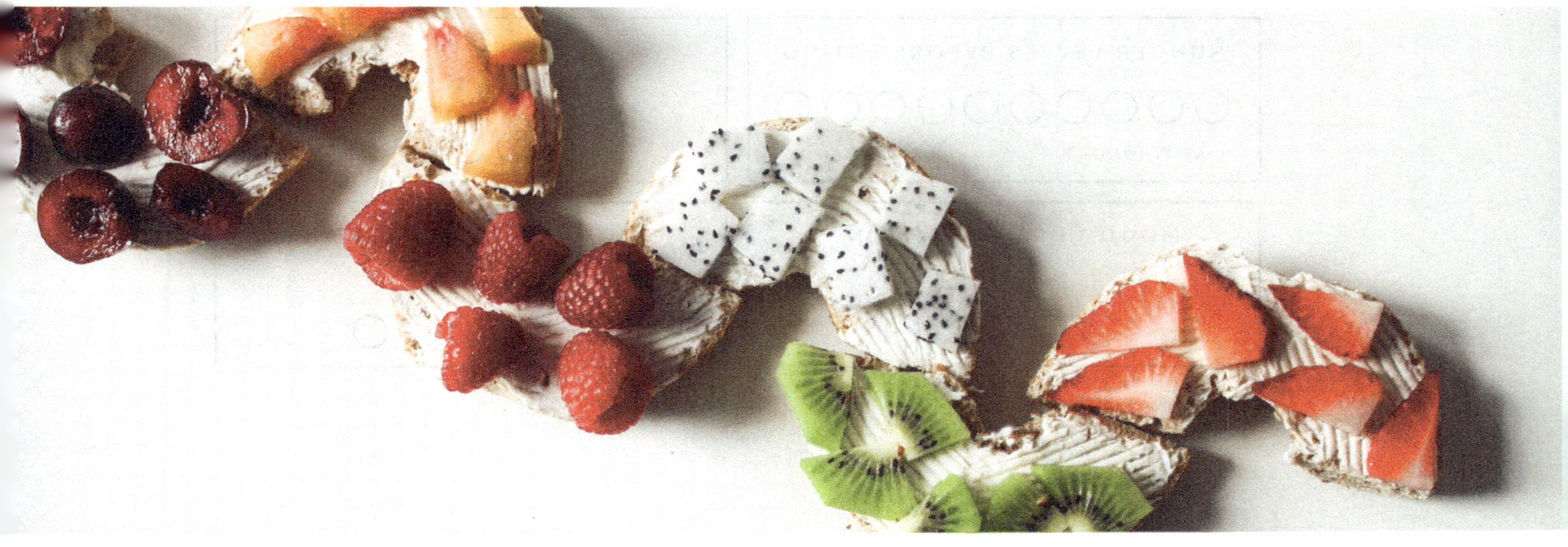

Food & Drink Removal

3 WEEK

Day 4

Remove specific foods and drinks identified in Week 2 from your diet and observe any changes in your symptoms.

BREAKFAST

LUNCH

DINNER

SNACKS

DRINKS CONSUMED *(INCLUDING ALCOHOL)*

SUPPLEMENTS/MEDICATIONS TAKEN

HUNGER LEVELS BEFORE EATING

○ ○ ○ ○ ○ ○ ○ ○ ○ ○

1- NOT HUNGRY *10 - RAVENOUS*

MOOD BEFORE EATING

○ ○ ○ ○ ○

MOOD 1 HR AFTER EATING

○ ○ ○ ○ ○

MOOD 3 HRS AFTER EATING

○ ○ ○ ○ ○

BREAKFAST

LUNCH

DINNER

SNACKS

DRINKS CONSUMED *(INCLUDING ALCOHOL)*

SUPPLEMENTS/MEDICATIONS TAKEN

HUNGER LEVELS BEFORE EATING

○ ○ ○ ○ ○ ○ ○ ○ ○ ○

1- NOT HUNGRY *10 - RAVENOUS*

MOOD BEFORE EATING

○ ○ ○ ○ ○

MOOD 1 HR AFTER EATING

○ ○ ○ ○ ○

MOOD 3 HRS AFTER EATING

○ ○ ○ ○ ○

3 WEEK

Food & Drink Removal

Remove specific foods and drinks identified in Week 2 from your diet and observe any changes in your symptoms.

Day 4

BREAKFAST

LUNCH

DINNER

SNACKS

DRINKS CONSUMED *(INCLUDING ALCOHOL)*

SUPPLEMENTS/MEDICATIONS TAKEN

HUNGER LEVELS BEFORE EATING

1- NOT HUNGRY *10 - RAVENOUS*

MOOD BEFORE EATING

MOOD 1 HR AFTER EATING

MOOD 3 HRS AFTER EATING

BREAKFAST

LUNCH

DINNER

SNACKS

DRINKS CONSUMED *(INCLUDING ALCOHOL)*

SUPPLEMENTS/MEDICATIONS TAKEN

HUNGER LEVELS BEFORE EATING

1- NOT HUNGRY *10 - RAVENOUS*

MOOD BEFORE EATING

MOOD 1 HR AFTER EATING

MOOD 3 HRS AFTER EATING

3
WEEK

Food & Drink Removal

Remove specific foods and drinks identified in Week 2 from your diet and observe any changes in your symptoms.

Observations

- [ ] Bloating
- [ ] Energy Spike
- [ ] Irritability
- [ ] Headache
- [ ] Skin Reaction
- [ ] Nausea
- [ ] Vomiting
- [ ] Constipation
- [ ] Diarrhea
- [ ] Gas
- [ ] Other *(space for them to explain)*

Perimenopausal/Menopausal Symptoms

Symptoms Experienced

- [ ] Hot Flashes
- [ ] Sweating
- [ ] Night Sweats
- [ ] Anxiety
- [ ] Bloating
- [ ] Fatigue
- [ ] Gas
- [ ] Brain Fog
- [ ] Poor Concentration
- [ ] Mood Swings
- [ ] Cravings
- [ ] Sleep Disturbances
- [ ] Vaginal Dryness
- [ ] Headache
- [ ] Other (please explain)

- [ ] Mild
- [ ] Moderate
- [ ] Severe

Duration of Symptoms

- [ ] 5 Mins
- [ ] 15 Mins
- [ ] 1 Hour

New Symptoms:

Please explain

Observations:

Please explain

3
WEEK

Food & Drink Removal

Remove specific foods and drinks identified in Week 2 from your diet and observe any changes in your symptoms.

Physical Activity

Type of Activity:

Duration:

Intensity:

☐ Low ☐ Moderate ☐ High

Sleep

Quality of Sleep:

☐ Excellent ☐ Poor
☐ Good ☐ Very Poor
☐ Fair

Hours Slept:

____
____
____

Support System:

Stress Management Techniques:

Water Intake Tracker:

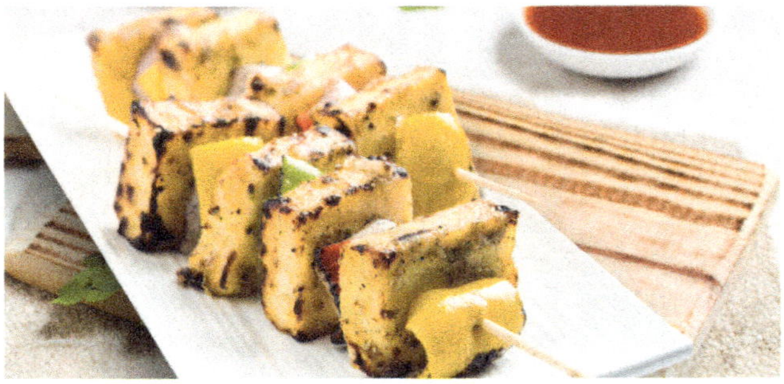

Overall Observations for the Day:

3 WEEK

Food & Drink Removal

Breastfeeding / Pumping Information

TIME	FEEDING / PUMPING		SLEEP OR ACTIVITY	BABY TOILETING	
	DURATION (Feeding)	AMOUNT (Bottle/ Pump)		PEE	POOP

Feelings & Observations

3
WEEK

Evening Reflections

Declutter Your Mind

As the day ends, take a moment to ***reflect on your day,*** and use this space to ***declutter your mind.*** Jot down your thoughts, feelings, and any moments that stood out. ***Often referred to as a "brain dump,"*** it's a method to understand, process, and release lingering thoughts that have built up throughout the day. Doing so will help to reduce stress and pave the way for a more peaceful night.

Thoughts/feelings

Use this space to let go of everything on your mind and write down your thoughts and feelings (from fleeting thoughts to deepest emotions). Writing them down without feeling "judged" helps you understand your feelings and prevents nighttime overthinking as you drift off to sleep.

Highlights and Today's Wins

What made you smile, feel proud, or brought you a sense of accomplishment today? Celebrate even the smallest wins and what you are especially thankful for here.

3
WEEK

Evening Reflections

Declutter Your Mind

Steps to Prepare For Tomorrow

Consider today's challenges. Which moments or areas is there room for growth or change? What steps can you take for a "better" tomorrow?

Rate Your Day

How would you describe your day on a scale of 1 to 10?
Use the emojis below as a guide, with 1 representing a difficult day and 10 symbolising an exceptional one...

1	2	3	4	5	6	7	8	9	10

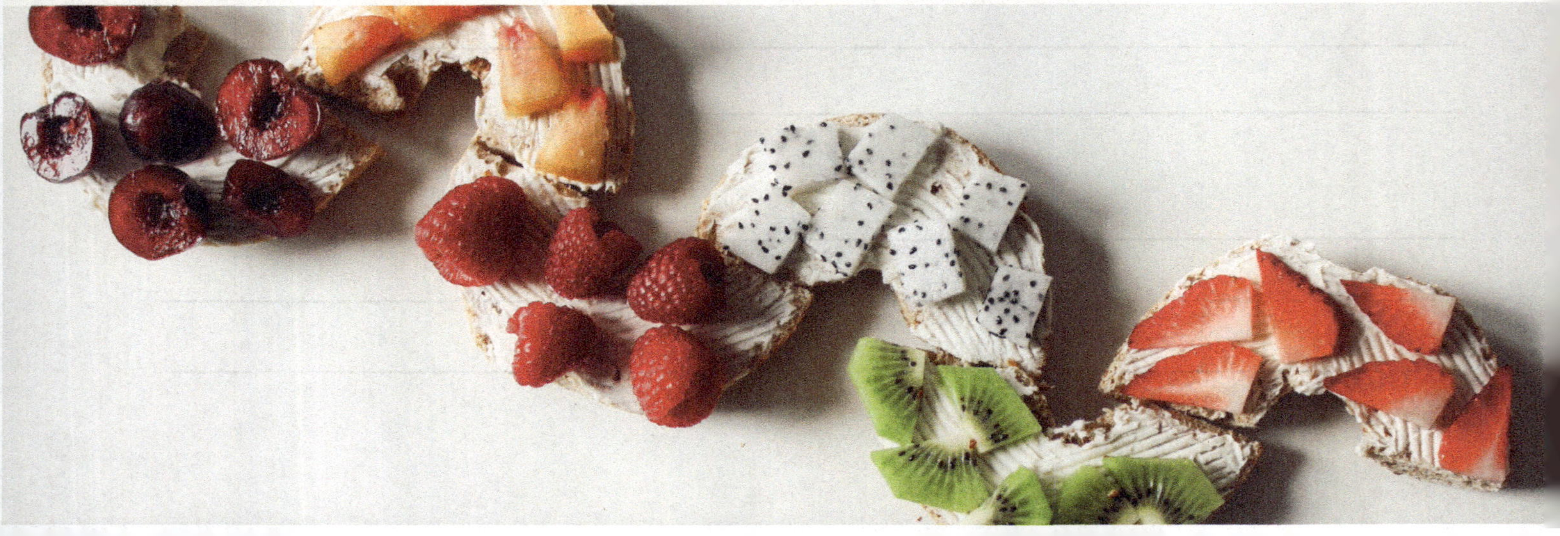

3 WEEK

Food & Drink Removal

Day 5

Remove specific foods and drinks identified in Week 2 from your diet and observe any changes in your symptoms.

BREAKFAST

LUNCH

DINNER

SNACKS

DRINKS CONSUMED *(INCLUDING ALCOHOL)*

SUPPLEMENTS/MEDICATIONS TAKEN

HUNGER LEVELS BEFORE EATING

○ ○ ○ ○ ○ ○ ○ ○ ○ ○

1- NOT HUNGRY *10 - RAVENOUS*

MOOD BEFORE EATING

○ ○ ○ ○ ○

MOOD 1 HR AFTER EATING

○ ○ ○ ○ ○

MOOD 3 HRS AFTER EATING

○ ○ ○ ○ ○

BREAKFAST

LUNCH

DINNER

SNACKS

DRINKS CONSUMED *(INCLUDING ALCOHOL)*

SUPPLEMENTS/MEDICATIONS TAKEN

HUNGER LEVELS BEFORE EATING

○ ○ ○ ○ ○ ○ ○ ○ ○ ○

1- NOT HUNGRY *10 - RAVENOUS*

MOOD BEFORE EATING

○ ○ ○ ○ ○

MOOD 1 HR AFTER EATING

○ ○ ○ ○ ○

MOOD 3 HRS AFTER EATING

○ ○ ○ ○ ○

3 WEEK

Food & Drink Removal

Day 5

Remove specific foods and drinks identified in Week 2 from your diet and observe any changes in your symptoms.

BREAKFAST

LUNCH

DINNER

SNACKS

DRINKS CONSUMED *(INCLUDING ALCOHOL)*

SUPPLEMENTS/MEDICATIONS TAKEN

HUNGER LEVELS BEFORE EATING

○ ○ ○ ○ ○ ○ ○ ○ ○ ○

1- NOT HUNGRY *10 - RAVENOUS*

MOOD BEFORE EATING

○ ○ ○ ○ ○

MOOD 1 HR AFTER EATING

○ ○ ○ ○ ○

MOOD 3 HRS AFTER EATING

○ ○ ○ ○ ○

BREAKFAST

LUNCH

DINNER

SNACKS

DRINKS CONSUMED *(INCLUDING ALCOHOL)*

SUPPLEMENTS/MEDICATIONS TAKEN

HUNGER LEVELS BEFORE EATING

○ ○ ○ ○ ○ ○ ○ ○ ○ ○

1- NOT HUNGRY *10 - RAVENOUS*

MOOD BEFORE EATING

○ ○ ○ ○ ○

MOOD 1 HR AFTER EATING

○ ○ ○ ○ ○

MOOD 3 HRS AFTER EATING

○ ○ ○ ○ ○

3
WEEK

Food & Drink Removal

Remove specific foods and drinks identified in Week 2 from your diet and observe any changes in your symptoms.

Observations

- [ ] Bloating
- [ ] Nausea
- [ ] Energy Spike
- [ ] Vomiting
- [ ] Irritability
- [ ] Constipation
- [ ] Headache
- [ ] Diarrhea
- [ ] Skin Reaction
- [ ] Gas
- [ ] Other *(space for them to explain)*

Perimenopausal/Menopausal Symptoms

Symptoms Experienced

- [ ] Hot Flashes
- [ ] Poor Concentration
- [ ] Sweating
- [ ] Mood Swings
- [ ] Night Sweats
- [ ] Cravings
- [ ] Anxiety
- [ ] Sleep Disturbances
- [ ] Bloating
- [ ] Vaginal Dryness
- [ ] Fatigue
- [ ] Headache
- [ ] Gas
- [ ] Other (please explain)
- [ ] Brain Fog

- [ ] Mild
- [ ] Moderate
- [ ] Severe

Duration of Symptoms

- [ ] 5 Mins
- [ ] 15 Mins
- [ ] 1 Hour

New Symptoms:

Please explain

Observations:

Please explain

3
WEEK

Food & Drink Removal

Remove specific foods and drinks identified in Week 2 from your diet and observe any changes in your symptoms.

Physical Activity

Type of Activity:

Duration:

Intensity:

☐ Low ☐ Moderate ☐ High

Sleep

Quality of Sleep:

☐ Excellent ☐ Poor
☐ Good ☐ Very Poor
☐ Fair

Hours Slept:

Support System:

Stress Management Techniques:

Water Intake Tracker:

Overall Observations for the Day:

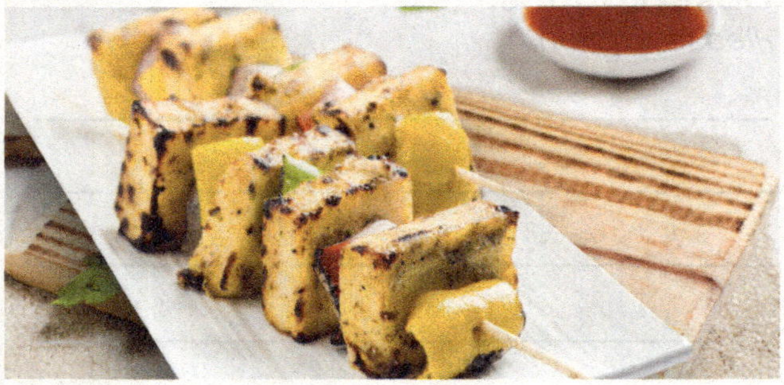

3
WEEK

Food & Drink Removal

Breastfeeding / Pumping Information

TIME	FEEDING / PUMPING		SLEEP OR ACTIVITY	BABY TOILETING	
	DURATION (Feeding)	AMOUNT (Bottle/ Pump)		PEE	POOP

Feelings & Observations

3
WEEK

Evening Reflections
Declutter Your Mind

As the day ends, take a moment to ***reflect on your day,*** and use this space to ***declutter your mind.*** Jot down your thoughts, feelings, and any moments that stood out. ***Often referred to as a "brain dump,"*** it's a method to understand, process, and release lingering thoughts that have built up throughout the day. Doing so will help to reduce stress and pave the way for a more peaceful night.

Thoughts/feelings

Use this space to let go of everything on your mind and write down your thoughts and feelings (from fleeting thoughts to deepest emotions). Writing them down without feeling "judged" helps you understand your feelings and prevents nighttime overthinking as you drift off to sleep.

Highlights and Today's Wins

What made you smile, feel proud, or brought you a sense of accomplishment today? Celebrate even the smallest wins and what you are especially thankful for here.

3
WEEK

Evening Reflections

Declutter Your Mind

Steps to Prepare For Tomorrow

Consider today's challenges. Which moments or areas is there room for growth or change? What steps can you take for a "better" tomorrow?

Rate Your Day

How would you describe your day on a scale of 1 to 10?
Use the emojis below as a guide, with 1 representing a difficult day and 10 symbolising an exceptional one...

1	2	3	4	5	6	7	8	9	10

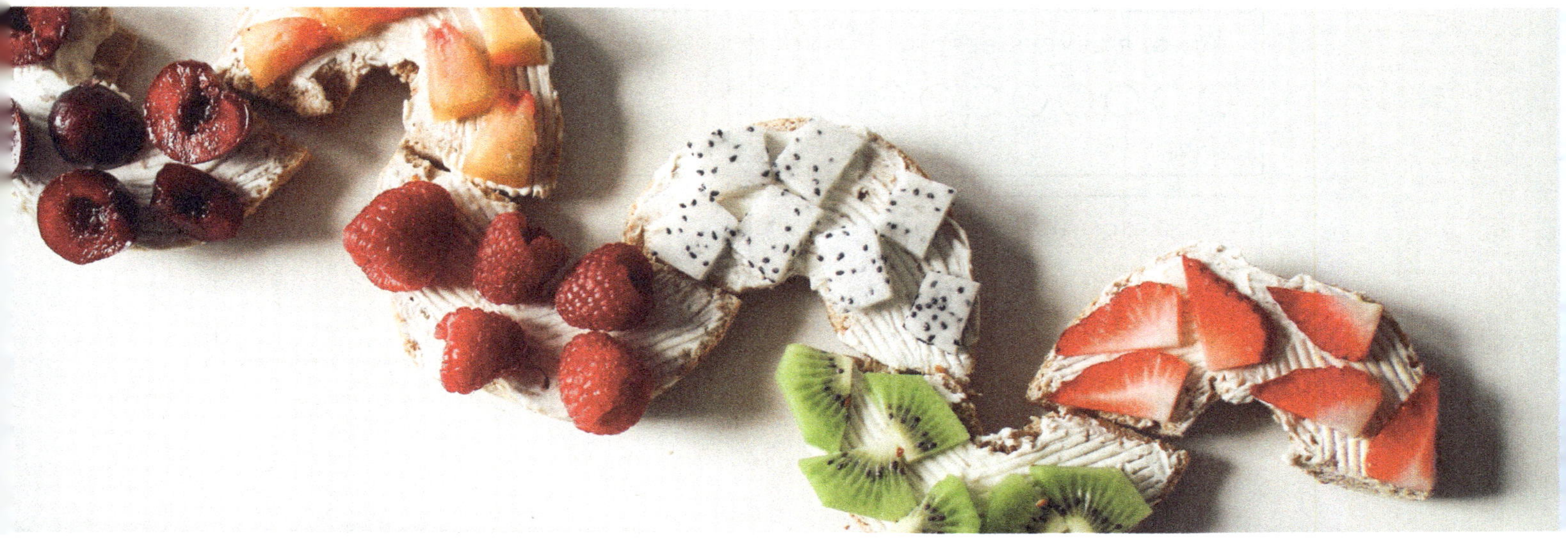

3 WEEK

Food & Drink Removal

Day 6

Remove specific foods and drinks identified in Week 2 from your diet and observe any changes in your symptoms.

BREAKFAST

LUNCH

DINNER

SNACKS

DRINKS CONSUMED *(INCLUDING ALCOHOL)*

SUPPLEMENTS/MEDICATIONS TAKEN

HUNGER LEVELS BEFORE EATING

○○○○○○○○○○

1- NOT HUNGRY *10 - RAVENOUS*

MOOD BEFORE EATING

○○○○○

MOOD 1 HR AFTER EATING

○○○○○

MOOD 3 HRS AFTER EATING

○○○○○

BREAKFAST

LUNCH

DINNER

SNACKS

DRINKS CONSUMED *(INCLUDING ALCOHOL)*

SUPPLEMENTS/MEDICATIONS TAKEN

HUNGER LEVELS BEFORE EATING

○○○○○○○○○○

1- NOT HUNGRY *10 - RAVENOUS*

MOOD BEFORE EATING

○○○○○

MOOD 1 HR AFTER EATING

○○○○○

MOOD 3 HRS AFTER EATING

○○○○○

3 WEEK

Food & Drink Removal

Remove specific foods and drinks identified in Week 2 from your diet and observe any changes in your symptoms.

Day 6

BREAKFAST

LUNCH

DINNER

SNACKS

DRINKS CONSUMED *(INCLUDING ALCOHOL)*

SUPPLEMENTS/MEDICATIONS TAKEN

HUNGER LEVELS BEFORE EATING

○ ○ ○ ○ ○ ○ ○ ○ ○ ○

1- NOT HUNGRY *10 - RAVENOUS*

MOOD BEFORE EATING

○ ○ ○ ○ ○

MOOD 1 HR AFTER EATING

○ ○ ○ ○ ○

MOOD 3 HRS AFTER EATING

○ ○ ○ ○ ○

BREAKFAST

LUNCH

DINNER

SNACKS

DRINKS CONSUMED *(INCLUDING ALCOHOL)*

SUPPLEMENTS/MEDICATIONS TAKEN

HUNGER LEVELS BEFORE EATING

○ ○ ○ ○ ○ ○ ○ ○ ○ ○

1- NOT HUNGRY *10 - RAVENOUS*

MOOD BEFORE EATING

○ ○ ○ ○ ○

MOOD 1 HR AFTER EATING

○ ○ ○ ○ ○

MOOD 3 HRS AFTER EATING

○ ○ ○ ○ ○

3
WEEK

Food & Drink Removal

Remove specific foods and drinks identified in Week 2 from your diet and observe any changes in your symptoms.

Observations

- [ ] Bloating
- [ ] Nausea
- [ ] Energy Spike
- [ ] Vomiting
- [ ] Irritability
- [ ] Constipation
- [ ] Headache
- [ ] Diarrhea
- [ ] Skin Reaction
- [ ] Gas
- [ ] Other *(space for them to explain)*

Perimenopausal/Menopausal Symptoms

Symptoms Experienced

- [ ] Hot Flashes
- [ ] Poor Concentration
- [ ] Sweating
- [ ] Mood Swings
- [ ] Night Sweats
- [ ] Cravings
- [ ] Anxiety
- [ ] Sleep Disturbances
- [ ] Bloating
- [ ] Vaginal Dryness
- [ ] Fatigue
- [ ] Headache
- [ ] Gas
- [ ] Other (please explain)
- [ ] Brain Fog

- [ ] Mild
- [ ] Moderate
- [ ] Severe

Duration of Symptoms

- [ ] 5 Mins
- [ ] 15 Mins
- [ ] 1 Hour

New Symptoms:
Please explain

Observations:
Please explain

3
WEEK

Food & Drink Removal

Remove specific foods and drinks identified in Week 2 from your diet and observe any changes in your symptoms.

Physical Activity

Type of Activity:

Duration:

Intensity:

☐ Low ☐ Moderate ☐ High

Sleep

Quality of Sleep:

☐ Excellent ☐ Poor
☐ Good ☐ Very Poor
☐ Fair

Hours Slept:

____

____

____

Support System:

Stress Management Techniques:

Water Intake Tracker:

💧 💧 💧 💧 💧 💧 💧 💧

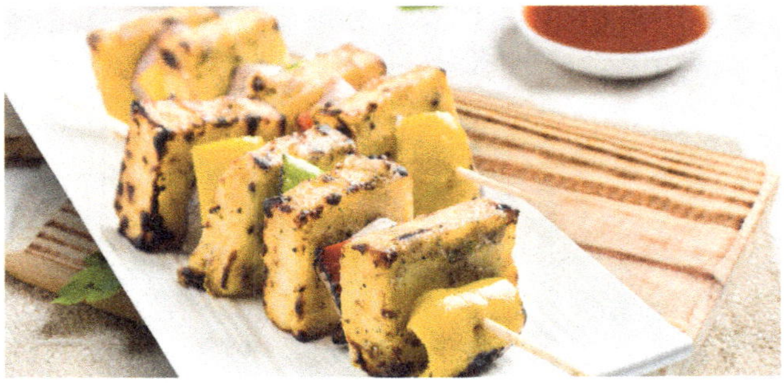

Overall Observations for the Day:

3
WEEK

Food & Drink Removal

Breastfeeding / Pumping Information

TIME	FEEDING / PUMPING		SLEEP OR ACTIVITY	BABY TOILETING	
	DURATION (Feeding)	AMOUNT (Bottle/ Pump)		PEE	POOP

Feelings & Observations

3
WEEK

Evening Reflections

Declutter Your Mind

As the day ends, take a moment to ***reflect on your day,*** and use this space to ***declutter your mind.*** Jot down your thoughts, feelings, and any moments that stood out. ***Often referred to as a "brain dump,"*** it's a method to understand, process, and release lingering thoughts that have built up throughout the day. Doing so will help to reduce stress and pave the way for a more peaceful night.

Thoughts/feelings

Use this space to let go of everything on your mind and write down your thoughts and feelings (from fleeting thoughts to deepest emotions). Writing them down without feeling "judged" helps you understand your feelings and prevents nighttime overthinking as you drift off to sleep.

Highlights and Today's Wins

What made you smile, feel proud, or brought you a sense of accomplishment today? Celebrate even the smallest wins and what you are especially thankful for here.

3
WEEK

Evening Reflections

Declutter Your Mind

Steps to Prepare For Tomorrow

Consider today's challenges. Which moments or areas is there room for growth or change? What steps can you take for a "better" tomorrow?

Rate Your Day

How would you describe your day on a scale of 1 to 10?
Use the emojis below as a guide, with 1 representing a difficult day and 10 symbolising an exceptional one...

1	2	3	4	5	6	7	8	9	10

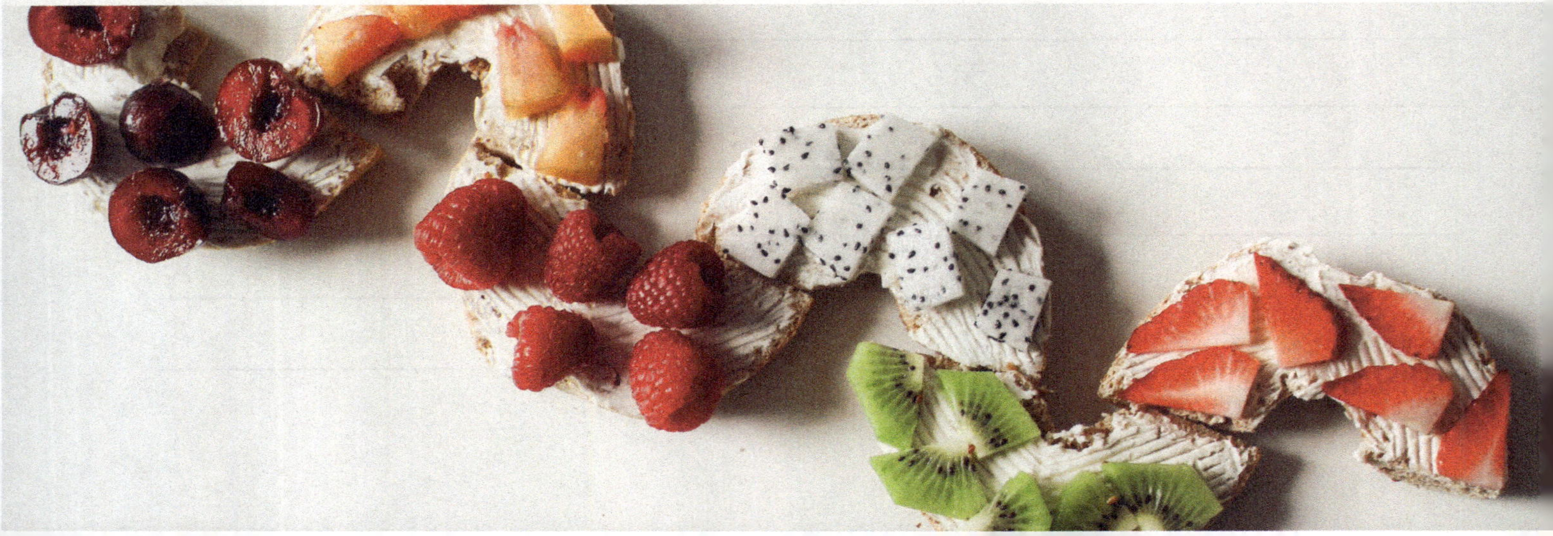

3
WEEK

Food & Drink Removal

Remove specific foods and drinks identified in Week 2 from your diet and observe any changes in your symptoms.

Day 7

BREAKFAST

LUNCH

DINNER

SNACKS

DRINKS CONSUMED *(INCLUDING ALCOHOL)*

SUPPLEMENTS/MEDICATIONS TAKEN

HUNGER LEVELS BEFORE EATING

○ ○ ○ ○ ○ ○ ○ ○ ○ ○

1- NOT HUNGRY *10 - RAVENOUS*

MOOD BEFORE EATING

○ ○ ○ ○ ○

MOOD 1 HR AFTER EATING

○ ○ ○ ○ ○

MOOD 3 HRS AFTER EATING

○ ○ ○ ○ ○

BREAKFAST

LUNCH

DINNER

SNACKS

DRINKS CONSUMED *(INCLUDING ALCOHOL)*

SUPPLEMENTS/MEDICATIONS TAKEN

HUNGER LEVELS BEFORE EATING

○ ○ ○ ○ ○ ○ ○ ○ ○ ○

1- NOT HUNGRY *10 - RAVENOUS*

MOOD BEFORE EATING

○ ○ ○ ○ ○

MOOD 1 HR AFTER EATING

○ ○ ○ ○ ○

MOOD 3 HRS AFTER EATING

○ ○ ○ ○ ○

Food & Drink Removal

3 WEEK

Day 7

Remove specific foods and drinks identified in Week 2 from your diet and observe any changes in your symptoms.

BREAKFAST

LUNCH

DINNER

SNACKS

DRINKS CONSUMED *(INCLUDING ALCOHOL)*

SUPPLEMENTS/MEDICATIONS TAKEN

HUNGER LEVELS BEFORE EATING

○ ○ ○ ○ ○ ○ ○ ○ ○ ○

1- NOT HUNGRY *10 - RAVENOUS*

MOOD BEFORE EATING

○ ○ ○ ○ ○

MOOD 1 HR AFTER EATING

○ ○ ○ ○ ○

MOOD 3 HRS AFTER EATING

○ ○ ○ ○ ○

BREAKFAST

LUNCH

DINNER

SNACKS

DRINKS CONSUMED *(INCLUDING ALCOHOL)*

SUPPLEMENTS/MEDICATIONS TAKEN

HUNGER LEVELS BEFORE EATING

○ ○ ○ ○ ○ ○ ○ ○ ○ ○

1- NOT HUNGRY *10 - RAVENOUS*

MOOD BEFORE EATING

○ ○ ○ ○ ○

MOOD 1 HR AFTER EATING

○ ○ ○ ○ ○

MOOD 3 HRS AFTER EATING

○ ○ ○ ○ ○

3
WEEK

Food & Drink Removal

Remove specific foods and drinks identified in Week 2 from your diet and observe any changes in your symptoms.

Observations

- [ ] Bloating
- [ ] Energy Spike
- [ ] Irritability
- [ ] Headache
- [ ] Skin Reaction
- [ ] Nausea
- [ ] Vomiting
- [ ] Constipation
- [ ] Diarrhea
- [ ] Gas
- [ ] Other *(space for them to explain)*

Perimenopausal/Menopausal Symptoms

Symptoms Experienced

- [ ] Hot Flashes
- [ ] Sweating
- [ ] Night Sweats
- [ ] Anxiety
- [ ] Bloating
- [ ] Fatigue
- [ ] Gas
- [ ] Brain Fog
- [ ] Poor Concentration
- [ ] Mood Swings
- [ ] Cravings
- [ ] Sleep Disturbances
- [ ] Vaginal Dryness
- [ ] Headache
- [ ] Other (please explain)

- [ ] Mild
- [ ] Moderate
- [ ] Severe

Duration of Symptoms

- [ ] 5 Mins
- [ ] 15 Mins
- [ ] 1 Hour

New Symptoms:

Please explain

Observations:

Please explain

3
WEEK

Food & Drink Removal

Remove specific foods and drinks identified in Week 2 from your diet and observe any changes in your symptoms.

Physical Activity

Type of Activity:

Duration:

Intensity:
☐ Low ☐ Moderate ☐ High

Sleep

Quality of Sleep:
☐ Excellent ☐ Poor
☐ Good ☐ Very Poor
☐ Fair

Hours Slept:

Support System:

Stress Management Techniques:

Water Intake Tracker:

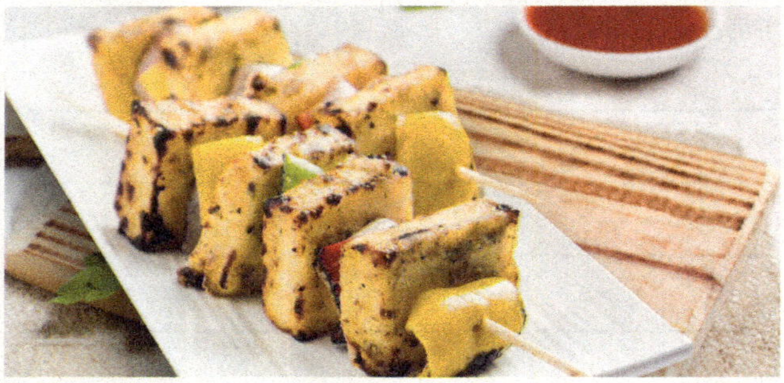

Overall Observations for the Day:

3 WEEK

Food & Drink Removal

Breastfeeding / Pumping Information

TIME	FEEDING / PUMPING		SLEEP OR ACTIVITY	BABY TOILETING	
	DURATION (Feeding)	AMOUNT (Bottle/ Pump)		PEE	POOP

Feelings & Observations

3
WEEK

Evening Reflections

Declutter Your Mind

As the day ends, take a moment to ***reflect on your day,*** and use this space to ***declutter your mind.*** Jot down your thoughts, feelings, and any moments that stood out. ***Often referred to as a "brain dump,"*** it's a method to understand, process, and release lingering thoughts that have built up throughout the day. Doing so will help to reduce stress and pave the way for a more peaceful night.

Thoughts/feelings

Use this space to let go of everything on your mind and write down your thoughts and feelings (from fleeting thoughts to deepest emotions). Writing them down without feeling "judged" helps you understand your feelings and prevents nighttime overthinking as you drift off to sleep.

Highlights and Today's Wins

What made you smile, feel proud, or brought you a sense of accomplishment today? Celebrate even the smallest wins and what you are especially thankful for here.

3 WEEK

Evening Reflections

Declutter Your Mind

Steps to Prepare For Tomorrow

Consider today's challenges. Which moments or areas is there room for growth or change? What steps can you take for a "better" tomorrow?

Rate Your Day

How would you describe your day on a scale of 1 to 10?
Use the emojis below as a guide, with 1 representing a difficult day and 10 symbolising an exceptional one...

1	2	3	4	5	6	7	8	9	10

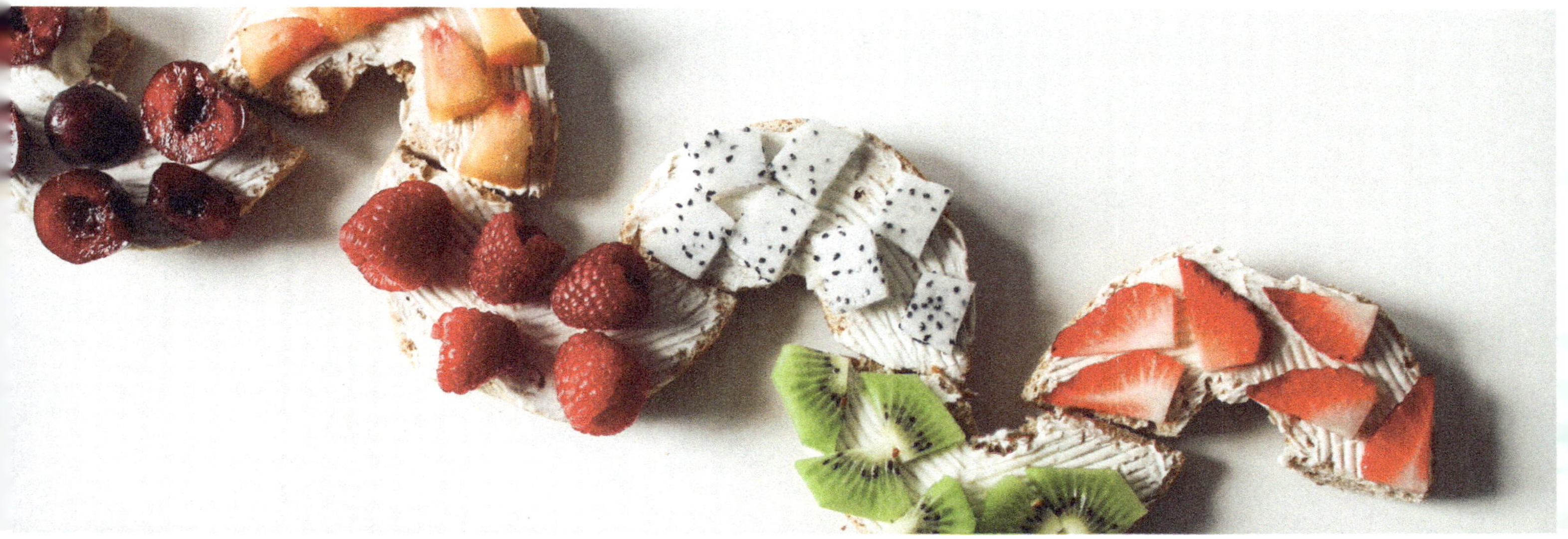

4
WEEK

Moving Forward

Symptom Management: Reflect on the dietary changes you have made over the past 3 weeks to help manage your symptoms and overall health moving forward.

Day 1

BREAKFAST

LUNCH

DINNER

SNACKS

DRINKS CONSUMED *(INCLUDING ALCOHOL)*

SUPPLEMENTS/MEDICATIONS TAKEN

HUNGER LEVELS BEFORE EATING

○ ○ ○ ○ ○ ○ ○ ○ ○ ○

1- NOT HUNGRY *10 - RAVENOUS*

MOOD BEFORE EATING

○ ○ ○ ○ ○

MOOD 1 HR AFTER EATING

○ ○ ○ ○ ○

MOOD 3 HRS AFTER EATING

○ ○ ○ ○ ○

BREAKFAST

LUNCH

DINNER

SNACKS

DRINKS CONSUMED *(INCLUDING ALCOHOL)*

SUPPLEMENTS/MEDICATIONS TAKEN

HUNGER LEVELS BEFORE EATING

○ ○ ○ ○ ○ ○ ○ ○ ○ ○

1- NOT HUNGRY *10 - RAVENOUS*

MOOD BEFORE EATING

○ ○ ○ ○ ○

MOOD 1 HR AFTER EATING

○ ○ ○ ○ ○

MOOD 3 HRS AFTER EATING

○ ○ ○ ○ ○

4
WEEK

Moving Forward

Day 1

Symptom Management: Reflect on the dietary changes you have made over the past 3 weeks to help manage your symptoms and overall health moving forward.

BREAKFAST

LUNCH

DINNER

SNACKS

DRINKS CONSUMED *(INCLUDING ALCOHOL)*

SUPPLEMENTS/MEDICATIONS TAKEN

HUNGER LEVELS BEFORE EATING

○ ○ ○ ○ ○ ○ ○ ○ ○ ○

1- NOT HUNGRY *10 - RAVENOUS*

MOOD BEFORE EATING

○ ○ ○ ○ ○

MOOD 1 HR AFTER EATING

○ ○ ○ ○ ○

MOOD 3 HRS AFTER EATING

○ ○ ○ ○ ○

BREAKFAST

LUNCH

DINNER

SNACKS

DRINKS CONSUMED *(INCLUDING ALCOHOL)*

SUPPLEMENTS/MEDICATIONS TAKEN

HUNGER LEVELS BEFORE EATING

○ ○ ○ ○ ○ ○ ○ ○ ○ ○

1- NOT HUNGRY *10 - RAVENOUS*

MOOD BEFORE EATING

○ ○ ○ ○ ○

MOOD 1 HR AFTER EATING

○ ○ ○ ○ ○

MOOD 3 HRS AFTER EATING

○ ○ ○ ○ ○

4 WEEK

Moving Forward

Symptom Management: Reflect on the dietary changes you have made over the past 3 weeks to help manage your symptoms and overall health moving forward.

Observations

- [ ] Bloating
- [ ] Nausea
- [ ] Energy Spike
- [ ] Vomiting
- [ ] Irritability
- [ ] Constipation
- [ ] Headache
- [ ] Diarrhea
- [ ] Skin Reaction
- [ ] Gas
- [ ] Other *(space for them to explain)*

Perimenopausal/Menopausal Symptoms

Symptoms Experienced

- [ ] Hot Flashes
- [ ] Poor Concentration
- [ ] Sweating
- [ ] Mood Swings
- [ ] Night Sweats
- [ ] Cravings
- [ ] Anxiety
- [ ] Sleep Disturbances
- [ ] Bloating
- [ ] Vaginal Dryness
- [ ] Fatigue
- [ ] Headache
- [ ] Gas
- [ ] Other (please explain)
- [ ] Brain Fog

- [ ] Mild
- [ ] Moderate
- [ ] Severe

Duration of Symptoms

- [ ] 5 Mins
- [ ] 15 Mins
- [ ] 1 Hour

New Symptoms:

Please explain

Observations:

Please explain

4
WEEK

Moving Forward

Symptom Management: Reflect on the dietary changes you have made over the past 3 weeks to help manage your symptoms and overall health moving forward.

Physical Activity

Type of Activity:

Duration:

Intensity:

☐ Low ☐ Moderate ☐ High

Sleep

Quality of Sleep:

☐ Excellent ☐ Poor
☐ Good ☐ Very Poor
☐ Fair

Hours Slept:

____

____

____

Support System:

Stress Management Techniques:

Water Intake Tracker:

💧 💧 💧 💧 💧 💧 💧 💧

Overall Observations for the Day:

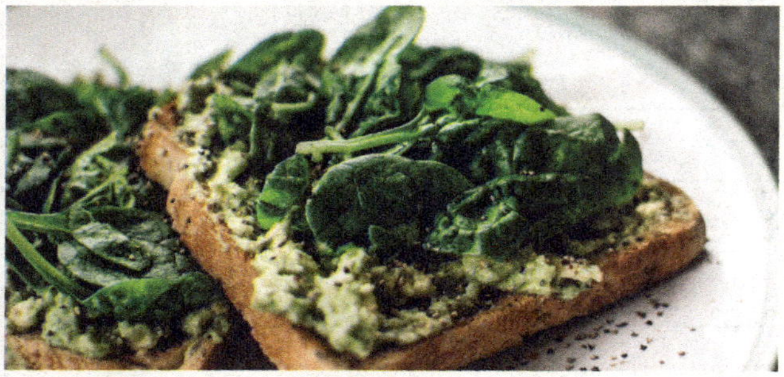

4 WEEK

Moving Forward

Symptom Management: Reflect on the dietary changes you have made over the past 3 weeks to help manage your symptoms and overall health moving forward.

Breastfeeding / Pumping Information

TIME	FEEDING / PUMPING		SLEEP OR ACTIVITY	BABY TOILETING	
	DURATION (Feeding)	AMOUNT (Bottle/ Pump)		PEE	POOP

Feelings & Observations

4 WEEK

Evening Reflections

Declutter Your Mind

As the day ends, take a moment to ***reflect on your day,*** and use this space to ***declutter your mind.*** Jot down your thoughts, feelings, and any moments that stood out. ***Often referred to as a "brain dump,"*** it's a method to understand, process, and release lingering thoughts that have built up throughout the day. Doing so will help to reduce stress and pave the way for a more peaceful night.

Thoughts/feelings

Use this space to let go of everything on your mind and write down your thoughts and feelings (from fleeting thoughts to deepest emotions). Writing them down without feeling "judged" helps you understand your feelings and prevents nighttime overthinking as you drift off to sleep.

Highlights and Today's Wins

What made you smile, feel proud, or brought you a sense of accomplishment today? Celebrate even the smallest wins and what you are especially thankful for here.

Evening Reflections

Declutter Your Mind

Steps to Prepare For Tomorrow

Consider today's challenges. Which moments or areas is there room for growth or change? What steps can you take for a "better" tomorrow?

Rate Your Day

How would you describe your day on a scale of 1 to 10?

Use the emojis below as a guide, with 1 representing a difficult day and 10 symbolising an exceptional one...

1	2	3	4	5	6	7	8	9	10

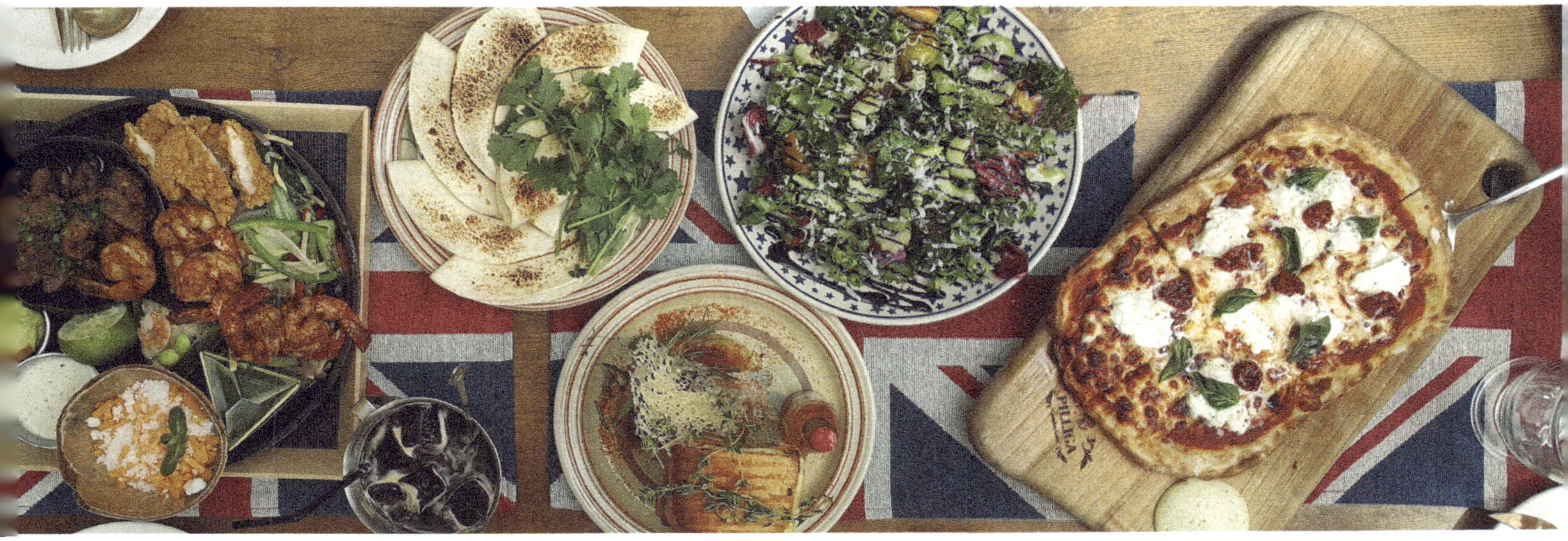

4
WEEK

Moving Forward

Day 2

Symptom Management: Reflect on the dietary changes you have made over the past 3 weeks to help manage your symptoms and overall health moving forward.

BREAKFAST

LUNCH

DINNER

SNACKS

DRINKS CONSUMED *(INCLUDING ALCOHOL)*

SUPPLEMENTS/MEDICATIONS TAKEN

HUNGER LEVELS BEFORE EATING

○ ○ ○ ○ ○ ○ ○ ○ ○ ○

1- NOT HUNGRY *10 - RAVENOUS*

MOOD BEFORE EATING

○ ○ ○ ○ ○

MOOD 1 HR AFTER EATING

○ ○ ○ ○ ○

MOOD 3 HRS AFTER EATING

○ ○ ○ ○ ○

BREAKFAST

LUNCH

DINNER

SNACKS

DRINKS CONSUMED *(INCLUDING ALCOHOL)*

SUPPLEMENTS/MEDICATIONS TAKEN

HUNGER LEVELS BEFORE EATING

○ ○ ○ ○ ○ ○ ○ ○ ○ ○

1- NOT HUNGRY *10 - RAVENOUS*

MOOD BEFORE EATING

○ ○ ○ ○ ○

MOOD 1 HR AFTER EATING

○ ○ ○ ○ ○

MOOD 3 HRS AFTER EATING

○ ○ ○ ○ ○

4 WEEK

Moving Forward

Day 2

Symptom Management: Reflect on the dietary changes you have made over the past 3 weeks to help manage your symptoms and overall health moving forward.

BREAKFAST

LUNCH

DINNER

SNACKS

DRINKS CONSUMED *(INCLUDING ALCOHOL)*

SUPPLEMENTS/MEDICATIONS TAKEN

HUNGER LEVELS BEFORE EATING

○ ○ ○ ○ ○ ○ ○ ○ ○ ○

1- NOT HUNGRY *10 - RAVENOUS*

MOOD BEFORE EATING

○ ○ ○ ○ ○

MOOD 1 HR AFTER EATING

○ ○ ○ ○ ○

MOOD 3 HRS AFTER EATING

○ ○ ○ ○ ○

BREAKFAST

LUNCH

DINNER

SNACKS

DRINKS CONSUMED *(INCLUDING ALCOHOL)*

SUPPLEMENTS/MEDICATIONS TAKEN

HUNGER LEVELS BEFORE EATING

○ ○ ○ ○ ○ ○ ○ ○ ○ ○

1- NOT HUNGRY *10 - RAVENOUS*

MOOD BEFORE EATING

○ ○ ○ ○ ○

MOOD 1 HR AFTER EATING

○ ○ ○ ○ ○

MOOD 3 HRS AFTER EATING

○ ○ ○ ○ ○

4 WEEK

Moving Forward

Symptom Management: Reflect on the dietary changes you have made over the past 3 weeks to help manage your symptoms and overall health moving forward.

Observations

- [ ] Bloating
- [ ] Energy Spike
- [ ] Irritability
- [ ] Headache
- [ ] Skin Reaction
- [ ] Nausea
- [ ] Vomiting
- [ ] Constipation
- [ ] Diarrhea
- [ ] Gas
- [ ] Other (*space for them to explain*)

Perimenopausal/Menopausal Symptoms

Symptoms Experienced

- [ ] Hot Flashes
- [ ] Sweating
- [ ] Night Sweats
- [ ] Anxiety
- [ ] Bloating
- [ ] Fatigue
- [ ] Gas
- [ ] Brain Fog
- [ ] Poor Concentration
- [ ] Mood Swings
- [ ] Cravings
- [ ] Sleep Disturbances
- [ ] Vaginal Dryness
- [ ] Headache
- [ ] Other (please explain)

- [ ] Mild
- [ ] Moderate
- [ ] Severe

Duration of Symptoms

- [ ] 5 Mins
- [ ] 15 Mins
- [ ] 1 Hour

New Symptoms:

Please explain

Observations:

Please explain

4
WEEK

Moving Forward

Symptom Management: Reflect on the dietary changes you have made over the past 3 weeks to help manage your symptoms and overall health moving forward.

Physical Activity

Type of Activity:

Duration:

Intensity:

☐ Low ☐ Moderate ☐ High

Sleep

Quality of Sleep:

☐ Excellent
☐ Good
☐ Fair
☐ Poor
☐ Very Poor

Hours Slept:

____

____

____

Support System:

Stress Management Techniques:

Water Intake Tracker:

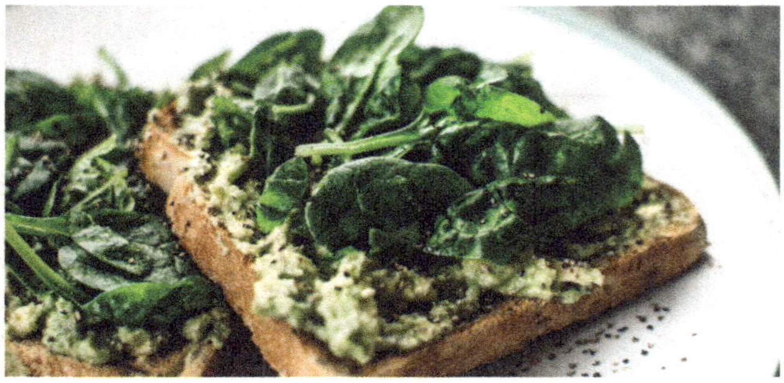

Overall Observations for the Day:

4
WEEK

Moving Forward

Symptom Management: Reflect on the dietary changes you have made over the past 3 weeks to help manage your symptoms and overall health moving forward.

Breastfeeding / Pumping Information

TIME	FEEDING / PUMPING		SLEEP OR ACTIVITY	BABY TOILETING	
	DURATION (Feeding)	AMOUNT (Bottle/ Pump)		PEE	POOP

Feelings & Observations

4
WEEK

Evening Reflections

Declutter Your Mind

As the day ends, take a moment to ***reflect on your day,*** and use this space to ***declutter your mind.*** Jot down your thoughts, feelings, and any moments that stood out. ***Often referred to as a "brain dump,"*** it's a method to understand, process, and release lingering thoughts that have built up throughout the day. Doing so will help to reduce stress and pave the way for a more peaceful night.

Thoughts/feelings

Use this space to let go of everything on your mind and write down your thoughts and feelings (from fleeting thoughts to deepest emotions). Writing them down without feeling "judged" helps you understand your feelings and prevents nighttime overthinking as you drift off to sleep.

Highlights and Today's Wins

What made you smile, feel proud, or brought you a sense of accomplishment today? Celebrate even the smallest wins and what you are especially thankful for here.

Evening Reflections

4 WEEK

Declutter Your Mind

Steps to Prepare For Tomorrow

Consider today's challenges. Which moments or areas is there room for growth or change? What steps can you take for a "better" tomorrow?

Rate Your Day

How would you describe your day on a scale of 1 to 10?
Use the emojis below as a guide, with 1 representing a difficult day and 10 symbolising an exceptional one...

1	2	3	4	5	6	7	8	9	10

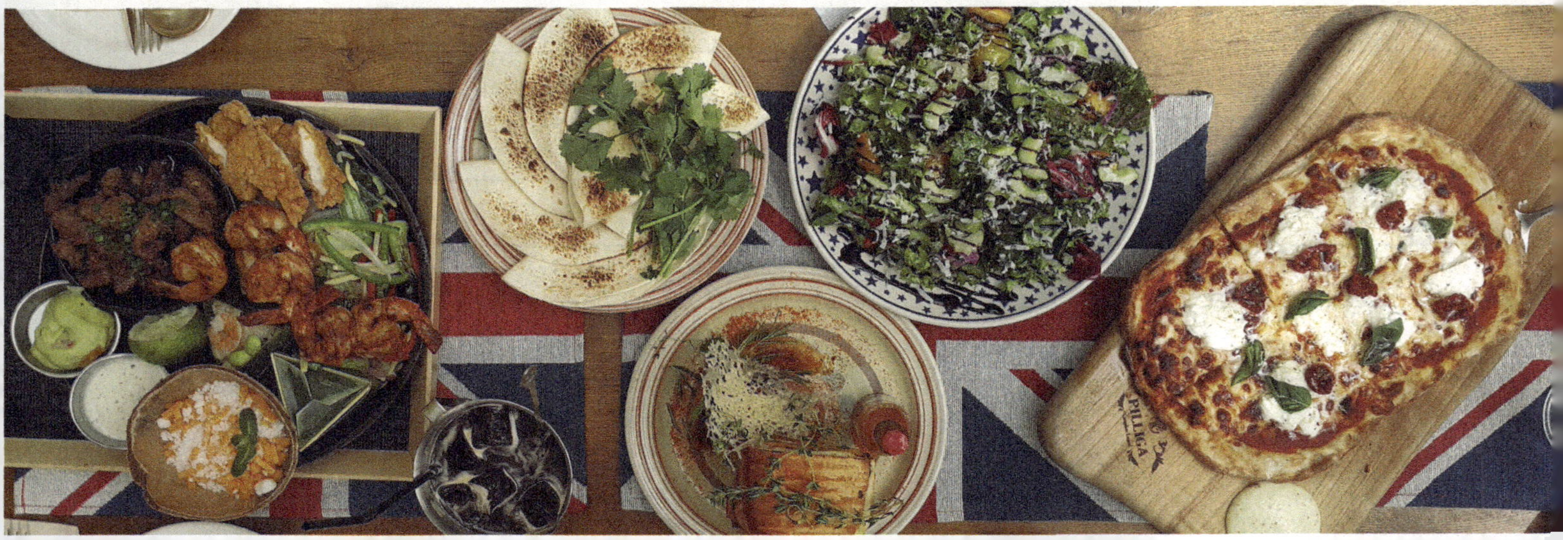

4
WEEK

Moving Forward

Symptom Management: Reflect on the dietary changes you have made over the past 3 weeks to help manage your symptoms and overall health moving forward.

Day 3

BREAKFAST

LUNCH

DINNER

SNACKS

DRINKS CONSUMED *(INCLUDING ALCOHOL)*

SUPPLEMENTS/MEDICATIONS TAKEN

HUNGER LEVELS BEFORE EATING

○ ○ ○ ○ ○ ○ ○ ○ ○ ○

1- NOT HUNGRY *10 - RAVENOUS*

MOOD BEFORE EATING

○ ○ ○ ○ ○

MOOD 1 HR AFTER EATING

○ ○ ○ ○ ○

MOOD 3 HRS AFTER EATING

○ ○ ○ ○ ○

BREAKFAST

LUNCH

DINNER

SNACKS

DRINKS CONSUMED *(INCLUDING ALCOHOL)*

SUPPLEMENTS/MEDICATIONS TAKEN

HUNGER LEVELS BEFORE EATING

○ ○ ○ ○ ○ ○ ○ ○ ○ ○

1- NOT HUNGRY *10 - RAVENOUS*

MOOD BEFORE EATING

○ ○ ○ ○ ○

MOOD 1 HR AFTER EATING

○ ○ ○ ○ ○

MOOD 3 HRS AFTER EATING

○ ○ ○ ○ ○

4
WEEK

Moving Forward

Symptom Management: Reflect on the dietary changes you have made over the past 3 weeks to help manage your symptoms and overall health moving forward.

Day 3

BREAKFAST

LUNCH

DINNER

SNACKS

DRINKS CONSUMED *(INCLUDING ALCOHOL)*

SUPPLEMENTS/MEDICATIONS TAKEN

HUNGER LEVELS BEFORE EATING

○ ○ ○ ○ ○ ○ ○ ○ ○ ○

1- NOT HUNGRY *10 - RAVENOUS*

MOOD BEFORE EATING

○ ○ ○ ○ ○

MOOD 1 HR AFTER EATING

○ ○ ○ ○ ○

MOOD 3 HRS AFTER EATING

○ ○ ○ ○ ○

BREAKFAST

LUNCH

DINNER

SNACKS

DRINKS CONSUMED *(INCLUDING ALCOHOL)*

SUPPLEMENTS/MEDICATIONS TAKEN

HUNGER LEVELS BEFORE EATING

○ ○ ○ ○ ○ ○ ○ ○ ○ ○

1- NOT HUNGRY *10 - RAVENOUS*

MOOD BEFORE EATING

○ ○ ○ ○ ○

MOOD 1 HR AFTER EATING

○ ○ ○ ○ ○

MOOD 3 HRS AFTER EATING

○ ○ ○ ○ ○

4 WEEK

Moving Forward

Symptom Management: Reflect on the dietary changes you have made over the past 3 weeks to help manage your symptoms and overall health moving forward.

Observations

____

____

____

____

____

____

- [ ] Bloating
- [ ] Energy Spike
- [ ] Irritability
- [ ] Headache
- [ ] Skin Reaction
- [ ] Nausea
- [ ] Vomiting
- [ ] Constipation
- [ ] Diarrhea
- [ ] Gas
- [ ] Other *(space for them to explain)*

____

Perimenopausal/Menopausal Symptoms

Symptoms Experienced

- [ ] Hot Flashes
- [ ] Sweating
- [ ] Night Sweats
- [ ] Anxiety
- [ ] Bloating
- [ ] Fatigue
- [ ] Gas
- [ ] Brain Fog
- [ ] Poor Concentration
- [ ] Mood Swings
- [ ] Cravings
- [ ] Sleep Disturbances
- [ ] Vaginal Dryness
- [ ] Headache
- [ ] Other (please explain)

____

- [ ] Mild
- [ ] Moderate
- [ ] Severe

Duration of Symptoms

____

____

____

____

____

____

____

- [ ] 5 Mins
- [ ] 15 Mins
- [ ] 1 Hour

New Symptoms:

Please explain

____

____

____

____

Observations:

Please explain

____

____

____

____

4
WEEK

Moving Forward

Symptom Management: Reflect on the dietary changes you have made over the past 3 weeks to help manage your symptoms and overall health moving forward.

Physical Activity

Type of Activity:

Duration:

Intensity:

☐ Low ☐ Moderate ☐ High

Sleep

Quality of Sleep:

☐ Excellent
☐ Poor
☐ Good
☐ Very Poor
☐ Fair

Hours Slept:

Support System:

Stress Management Techniques:

Water Intake Tracker:

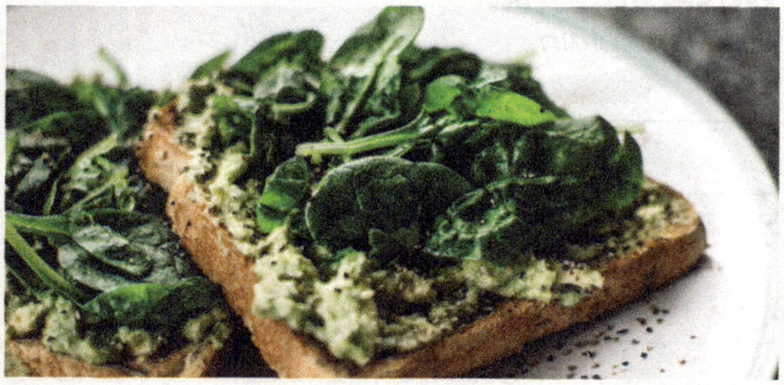

Overall Observations for the Day:

4
WEEK

Moving Forward

Symptom Management: Reflect on the dietary changes you have made over the past 3 weeks to help manage your symptoms and overall health moving forward.

Breastfeeding / Pumping Information

TIME	FEEDING / PUMPING		SLEEP OR ACTIVITY	BABY TOILETING	
	DURATION (Feeding)	AMOUNT (Bottle/ Pump)		PEE	POOP

Feelings & Observations

4
WEEK

Evening Reflections

Declutter Your Mind

As the day ends, take a moment to ***reflect on your day,*** and use this space to ***declutter your mind.*** Jot down your thoughts, feelings, and any moments that stood out. ***Often referred to as a "brain dump,"*** it's a method to understand, process, and release lingering thoughts that have built up throughout the day. Doing so will help to reduce stress and pave the way for a more peaceful night.

Thoughts/feelings

Use this space to let go of everything on your mind and write down your thoughts and feelings (from fleeting thoughts to deepest emotions). Writing them down without feeling "judged" helps you understand your feelings and prevents nighttime overthinking as you drift off to sleep.

Highlights and Today's Wins

What made you smile, feel proud, or brought you a sense of accomplishment today? Celebrate even the smallest wins and what you are especially thankful for here.

4 WEEK

Evening Reflections

Declutter Your Mind

Steps to Prepare For Tomorrow

Consider today's challenges. Which moments or areas is there room for growth or change? What steps can you take for a "better" tomorrow?

____

____

____

____

____

____

____

Rate Your Day

How would you describe your day on a scale of 1 to 10?

Use the emojis below as a guide, with 1 representing a difficult day and 10 symbolising an exceptional one...

☹									☺
1	2	3	4	5	6	7	8	9	10

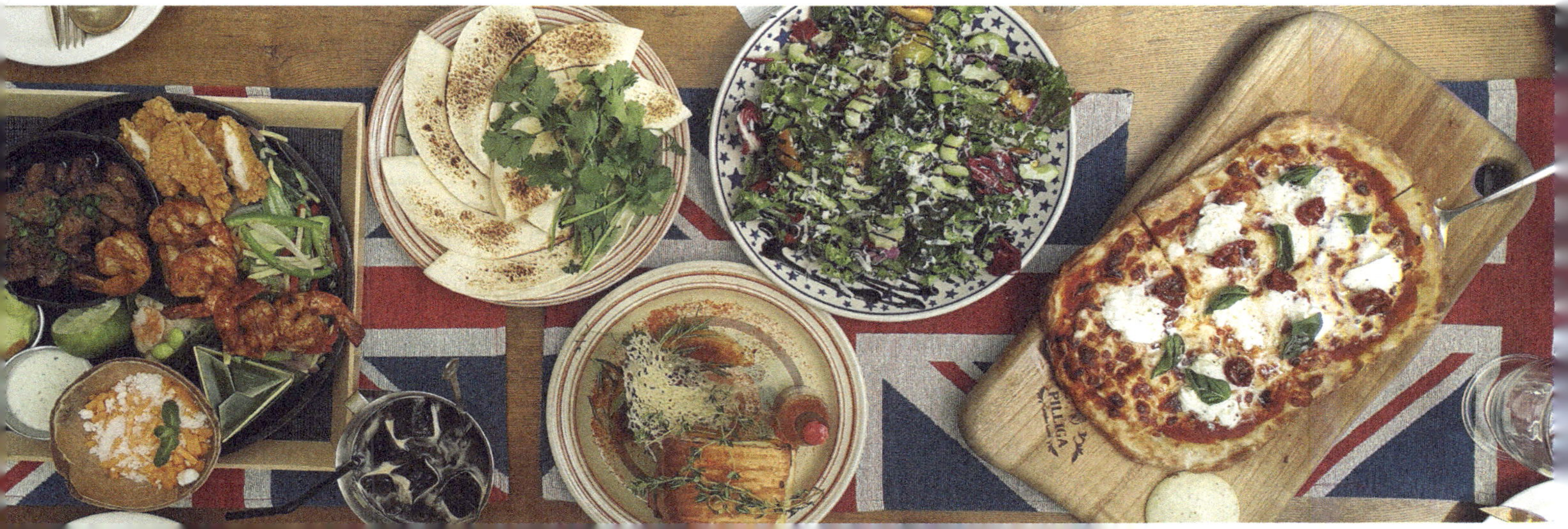

4
WEEK

Moving Forward

Day 4

Symptom Management: Reflect on the dietary changes you have made over the past 3 weeks to help manage your symptoms and overall health moving forward.

BREAKFAST

LUNCH

DINNER

SNACKS

DRINKS CONSUMED *(INCLUDING ALCOHOL)*

SUPPLEMENTS/MEDICATIONS TAKEN

HUNGER LEVELS BEFORE EATING

○ ○ ○ ○ ○ ○ ○ ○ ○ ○

1- NOT HUNGRY *10 - RAVENOUS*

MOOD BEFORE EATING

○ ○ ○ ○ ○

MOOD 1 HR AFTER EATING

○ ○ ○ ○ ○

MOOD 3 HRS AFTER EATING

○ ○ ○ ○ ○

BREAKFAST

LUNCH

DINNER

SNACKS

DRINKS CONSUMED *(INCLUDING ALCOHOL)*

SUPPLEMENTS/MEDICATIONS TAKEN

HUNGER LEVELS BEFORE EATING

○ ○ ○ ○ ○ ○ ○ ○ ○ ○

1- NOT HUNGRY *10 - RAVENOUS*

MOOD BEFORE EATING

○ ○ ○ ○ ○

MOOD 1 HR AFTER EATING

○ ○ ○ ○ ○

MOOD 3 HRS AFTER EATING

○ ○ ○ ○ ○

4 WEEK

Moving Forward

Symptom Management: Reflect on the dietary changes you have made over the past 3 weeks to help manage your symptoms and overall health moving forward.

Day 4

BREAKFAST

LUNCH

DINNER

SNACKS

DRINKS CONSUMED *(INCLUDING ALCOHOL)*

SUPPLEMENTS/MEDICATIONS TAKEN

HUNGER LEVELS BEFORE EATING

○ ○ ○ ○ ○ ○ ○ ○ ○ ○

1- NOT HUNGRY *10 - RAVENOUS*

MOOD BEFORE EATING

○ ○ ○ ○ ○

MOOD 1 HR AFTER EATING

○ ○ ○ ○ ○

MOOD 3 HRS AFTER EATING

○ ○ ○ ○ ○

BREAKFAST

LUNCH

DINNER

SNACKS

DRINKS CONSUMED *(INCLUDING ALCOHOL)*

SUPPLEMENTS/MEDICATIONS TAKEN

HUNGER LEVELS BEFORE EATING

○ ○ ○ ○ ○ ○ ○ ○ ○ ○

1- NOT HUNGRY *10 - RAVENOUS*

MOOD BEFORE EATING

○ ○ ○ ○ ○

MOOD 1 HR AFTER EATING

○ ○ ○ ○ ○

MOOD 3 HRS AFTER EATING

○ ○ ○ ○ ○

4 WEEK

Moving Forward

Symptom Management: Reflect on the dietary changes you have made over the past 3 weeks to help manage your symptoms and overall health moving forward.

Observations

____

____

____

____

____

____

- [ ] Bloating
- [ ] Energy Spike
- [ ] Irritability
- [ ] Headache
- [ ] Skin Reaction
- [ ] Nausea
- [ ] Vomiting
- [ ] Constipation
- [ ] Diarrhea
- [ ] Gas
- [ ] Other *(space for them to explain)*

____

Perimenopausal/Menopausal Symptoms

Symptoms Experienced

- [ ] Hot Flashes
- [ ] Sweating
- [ ] Night Sweats
- [ ] Anxiety
- [ ] Bloating
- [ ] Fatigue
- [ ] Gas
- [ ] Brain Fog
- [ ] Poor Concentration
- [ ] Mood Swings
- [ ] Cravings
- [ ] Sleep Disturbances
- [ ] Vaginal Dryness
- [ ] Headache
- [ ] Other (please explain)

____

- [ ] Mild
- [ ] Moderate
- [ ] Severe

Duration of Symptoms

____

____

____

____

____

____

____

- [ ] 5 Mins
- [ ] 15 Mins
- [ ] 1 Hour

New Symptoms:
Please explain

____

____

____

____

Observations:
Please explain

____

____

____

____

4 WEEK

Moving Forward

Symptom Management: Reflect on the dietary changes you have made over the past 3 weeks to help manage your symptoms and overall health moving forward.

Physical Activity

Type of Activity:

Duration:

Intensity:

☐ Low ☐ Moderate ☐ High

Sleep

Quality of Sleep:

☐ Excellent ☐ Poor
☐ Good ☐ Very Poor
☐ Fair

Hours Slept:

____

____

____

Support System:

Stress Management Techniques:

Water Intake Tracker:

💧 💧 💧 💧 💧 💧 💧 💧

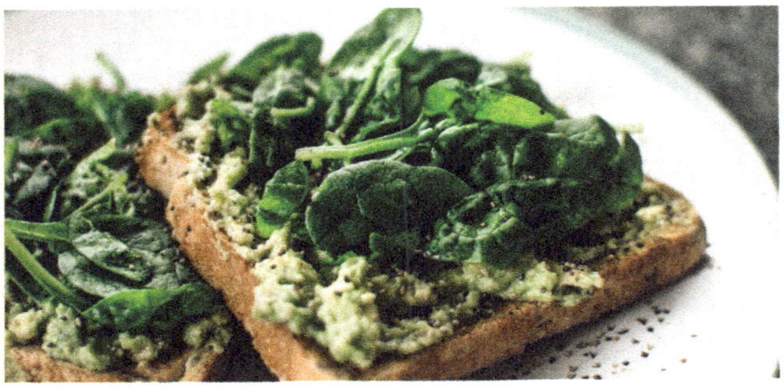

Overall Observations for the Day:

4
WEEK

Moving Forward

Symptom Management: Reflect on the dietary changes you have made over the past 3 weeks to help manage your symptoms and overall health moving forward.

Breastfeeding / Pumping Information

TIME	FEEDING / PUMPING		SLEEP OR ACTIVITY	BABY TOILETING	
	DURATION (Feeding)	AMOUNT (Bottle/ Pump)		PEE	POOP

Feelings & Observations

4
WEEK

Evening Reflections

Declutter Your Mind

As the day ends, take a moment to ***reflect on your day,*** and use this space to ***declutter your mind.*** Jot down your thoughts, feelings, and any moments that stood out. ***Often referred to as a "brain dump,"*** it's a method to understand, process, and release lingering thoughts that have built up throughout the day. Doing so will help to reduce stress and pave the way for a more peaceful night.

Thoughts/feelings

Use this space to let go of everything on your mind and write down your thoughts and feelings (from fleeting thoughts to deepest emotions). Writing them down without feeling "judged" helps you understand your feelings and prevents nighttime overthinking as you drift off to sleep.

Highlights and Today's Wins

What made you smile, feel proud, or brought you a sense of accomplishment today? Celebrate even the smallest wins and what you are especially thankful for here.

4 WEEK Evening Reflections

Declutter Your Mind

Steps to Prepare For Tomorrow

Consider today's challenges. Which moments or areas is there room for growth or change? What steps can you take for a "better" tomorrow?

Rate Your Day

How would you describe your day on a scale of 1 to 10?
Use the emojis below as a guide, with 1 representing a difficult day and 10 symbolising an exceptional one...

1	2	3	4	5	6	7	8	9	10

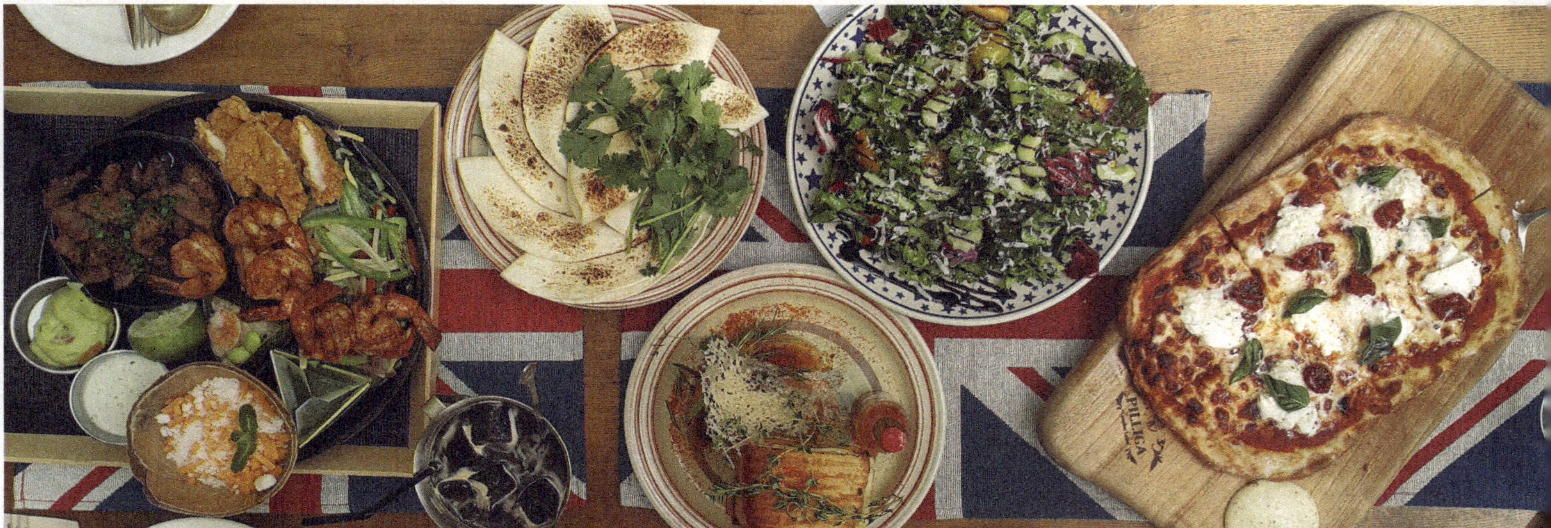

4
WEEK

Moving Forward

Symptom Management: Reflect on the dietary changes you have made over the past 3 weeks to help manage your symptoms and overall health moving forward.

Day 5

BREAKFAST

LUNCH

DINNER

SNACKS

DRINKS CONSUMED *(INCLUDING ALCOHOL)*

SUPPLEMENTS/MEDICATIONS TAKEN

HUNGER LEVELS BEFORE EATING

○ ○ ○ ○ ○ ○ ○ ○ ○ ○

1- NOT HUNGRY *10 - RAVENOUS*

MOOD BEFORE EATING

○ ○ ○ ○ ○

MOOD 1 HR AFTER EATING

○ ○ ○ ○ ○

MOOD 3 HRS AFTER EATING

○ ○ ○ ○ ○

BREAKFAST

LUNCH

DINNER

SNACKS

DRINKS CONSUMED *(INCLUDING ALCOHOL)*

SUPPLEMENTS/MEDICATIONS TAKEN

HUNGER LEVELS BEFORE EATING

○ ○ ○ ○ ○ ○ ○ ○ ○ ○

1- NOT HUNGRY *10 - RAVENOUS*

MOOD BEFORE EATING

○ ○ ○ ○ ○

MOOD 1 HR AFTER EATING

○ ○ ○ ○ ○

MOOD 3 HRS AFTER EATING

○ ○ ○ ○ ○

4
WEEK

Moving Forward

Day 5

Symptom Management: Reflect on the dietary changes you have made over the past 3 weeks to help manage your symptoms and overall health moving forward.

BREAKFAST

LUNCH

DINNER

SNACKS

DRINKS CONSUMED *(INCLUDING ALCOHOL)*

SUPPLEMENTS/MEDICATIONS TAKEN

HUNGER LEVELS BEFORE EATING

1- NOT HUNGRY *10 - RAVENOUS*

MOOD BEFORE EATING

MOOD 1 HR AFTER EATING

MOOD 3 HRS AFTER EATING

BREAKFAST

LUNCH

DINNER

SNACKS

DRINKS CONSUMED *(INCLUDING ALCOHOL)*

SUPPLEMENTS/MEDICATIONS TAKEN

HUNGER LEVELS BEFORE EATING

1- NOT HUNGRY *10 - RAVENOUS*

MOOD BEFORE EATING

MOOD 1 HR AFTER EATING

MOOD 3 HRS AFTER EATING

4
WEEK

Moving Forward

Symptom Management: Reflect on the dietary changes you have made over the past 3 weeks to help manage your symptoms and overall health moving forward.

Observations

- [ ] Bloating
- [ ] Energy Spike
- [ ] Irritability
- [ ] Headache
- [ ] Skin Reaction
- [ ] Nausea
- [ ] Vomiting
- [ ] Constipation
- [ ] Diarrhea
- [ ] Gas
- [ ] Other *(space for them to explain)*

Perimenopausal/Menopausal Symptoms

Symptoms Experienced

- [ ] Hot Flashes
- [ ] Sweating
- [ ] Night Sweats
- [ ] Anxiety
- [ ] Bloating
- [ ] Fatigue
- [ ] Gas
- [ ] Brain Fog
- [ ] Poor Concentration
- [ ] Mood Swings
- [ ] Cravings
- [ ] Sleep Disturbances
- [ ] Vaginal Dryness
- [ ] Headache
- [ ] Other (please explain)

- [ ] Mild
- [ ] Moderate
- [ ] Severe

Duration of Symptoms

- [ ] 5 Mins
- [ ] 15 Mins
- [ ] 1 Hour

New Symptoms:

Please explain

Observations:

Please explain

4 WEEK Moving Forward

Symptom Management: Reflect on the dietary changes you have made over the past 3 weeks to help manage your symptoms and overall health moving forward.

Physical Activity

Type of Activity:

Duration:

Intensity:

☐ Low ☐ Moderate ☐ High

Sleep

Quality of Sleep:

☐ Excellent
☐ Good
☐ Fair
☐ Poor
☐ Very Poor

Hours Slept:

Support System:

Stress Management Techniques:

Water Intake Tracker:

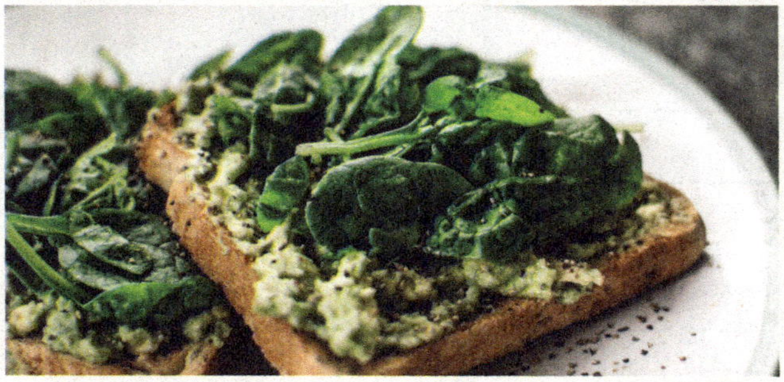

Overall Observations for the Day:

4 WEEK

Moving Forward

Symptom Management: Reflect on the dietary changes you have made over the past 3 weeks to help manage your symptoms and overall health moving forward.

Breastfeeding / Pumping Information

TIME	FEEDING / PUMPING		SLEEP OR ACTIVITY	BABY TOILETING	
	DURATION (Feeding)	AMOUNT (Bottle/ Pump)		PEE	POOP

Feelings & Observations

4 WEEK

Evening Reflections

Declutter Your Mind

As the day ends, take a moment to ***reflect on your day,*** and use this space to ***declutter your mind.*** Jot down your thoughts, feelings, and any moments that stood out. ***Often referred to as a "brain dump,"*** it's a method to understand, process, and release lingering thoughts that have built up throughout the day. Doing so will help to reduce stress and pave the way for a more peaceful night.

Thoughts/feelings

Use this space to let go of everything on your mind and write down your thoughts and feelings (from fleeting thoughts to deepest emotions). Writing them down without feeling "judged" helps you understand your feelings and prevents nighttime overthinking as you drift off to sleep.

Highlights and Today's Wins

What made you smile, feel proud, or brought you a sense of accomplishment today? Celebrate even the smallest wins and what you are especially thankful for here.

4
WEEK

Evening Reflections

Declutter Your Mind

Steps to Prepare For Tomorrow

Consider today's challenges. Which moments or areas is there room for growth or change? What steps can you take for a "better" tomorrow?

Rate Your Day

How would you describe your day on a scale of 1 to 10?
Use the emojis below as a guide, with 1 representing a difficult day and 10 symbolising an exceptional one...

1	2	3	4	5	6	7	8	9	10

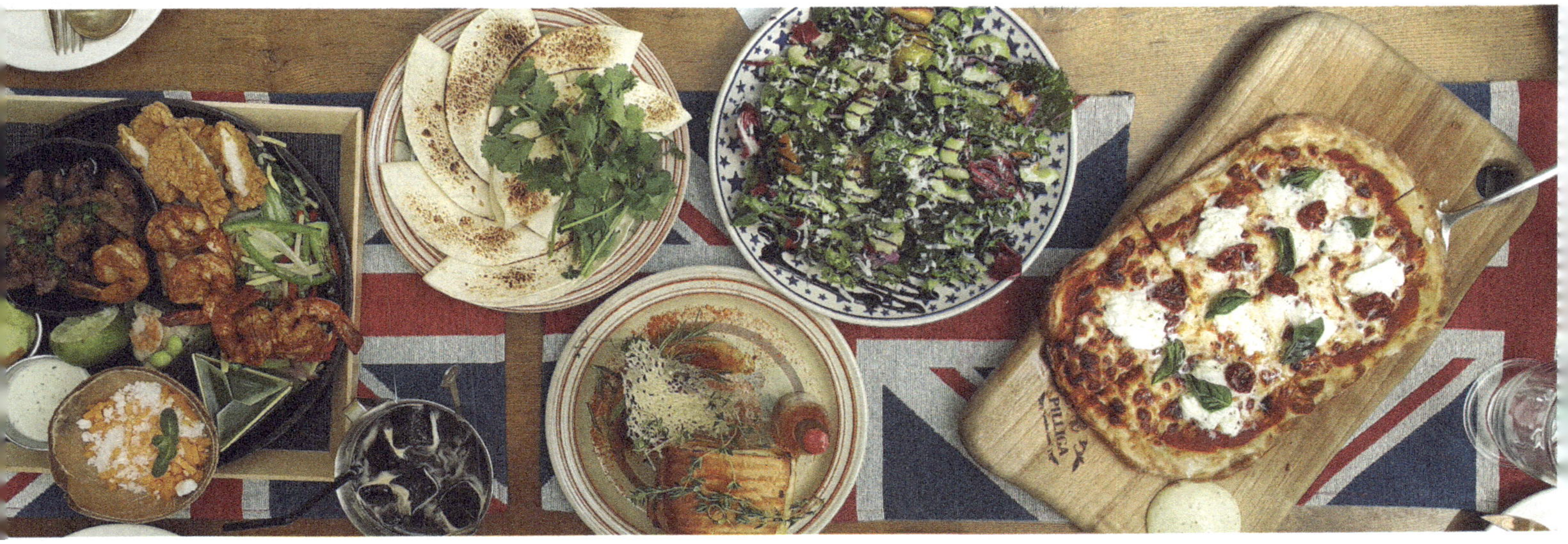

4 WEEK

Moving Forward

Day 6

Symptom Management: Reflect on the dietary changes you have made over the past 3 weeks to help manage your symptoms and overall health moving forward.

BREAKFAST

LUNCH

DINNER

SNACKS

DRINKS CONSUMED *(INCLUDING ALCOHOL)*

SUPPLEMENTS/MEDICATIONS TAKEN

HUNGER LEVELS BEFORE EATING

○ ○ ○ ○ ○ ○ ○ ○ ○ ○

1- NOT HUNGRY *10 - RAVENOUS*

MOOD BEFORE EATING

○ ○ ○ ○ ○

MOOD 1 HR AFTER EATING

○ ○ ○ ○ ○

MOOD 3 HRS AFTER EATING

○ ○ ○ ○ ○

BREAKFAST

LUNCH

DINNER

SNACKS

DRINKS CONSUMED *(INCLUDING ALCOHOL)*

SUPPLEMENTS/MEDICATIONS TAKEN

HUNGER LEVELS BEFORE EATING

○ ○ ○ ○ ○ ○ ○ ○ ○ ○

1- NOT HUNGRY *10 - RAVENOUS*

MOOD BEFORE EATING

○ ○ ○ ○ ○

MOOD 1 HR AFTER EATING

○ ○ ○ ○ ○

MOOD 3 HRS AFTER EATING

○ ○ ○ ○ ○

4 WEEK

Moving Forward

Day 6

Symptom Management: Reflect on the dietary changes you have made over the past 3 weeks to help manage your symptoms and overall health moving forward.

BREAKFAST

LUNCH

DINNER

SNACKS

DRINKS CONSUMED *(INCLUDING ALCOHOL)*

SUPPLEMENTS/MEDICATIONS TAKEN

HUNGER LEVELS BEFORE EATING

1- NOT HUNGRY *10 - RAVENOUS*

MOOD BEFORE EATING

MOOD 1 HR AFTER EATING

MOOD 3 HRS AFTER EATING

BREAKFAST

LUNCH

DINNER

SNACKS

DRINKS CONSUMED *(INCLUDING ALCOHOL)*

SUPPLEMENTS/MEDICATIONS TAKEN

HUNGER LEVELS BEFORE EATING

1- NOT HUNGRY *10 - RAVENOUS*

MOOD BEFORE EATING

MOOD 1 HR AFTER EATING

MOOD 3 HRS AFTER EATING

4
WEEK

Moving Forward

Symptom Management: Reflect on the dietary changes you have made over the past 3 weeks to help manage your symptoms and overall health moving forward.

Observations

- [ ] Bloating
- [ ] Energy Spike
- [ ] Irritability
- [ ] Headache
- [ ] Skin Reaction
- [ ] Nausea
- [ ] Vomiting
- [ ] Constipation
- [ ] Diarrhea
- [ ] Gas
- [ ] Other *(space for them to explain)*

Perimenopausal/Menopausal Symptoms

Symptoms Experienced

- [ ] Hot Flashes
- [ ] Sweating
- [ ] Night Sweats
- [ ] Anxiety
- [ ] Bloating
- [ ] Fatigue
- [ ] Gas
- [ ] Brain Fog
- [ ] Poor Concentration
- [ ] Mood Swings
- [ ] Cravings
- [ ] Sleep Disturbances
- [ ] Vaginal Dryness
- [ ] Headache
- [ ] Other (please explain)

- [ ] Mild
- [ ] Moderate
- [ ] Severe

Duration of Symptoms

- [ ] 5 Mins
- [ ] 15 Mins
- [ ] 1 Hour

New Symptoms:

Please explain

Observations:

Please explain

4
WEEK

Moving Forward

Symptom Management: Reflect on the dietary changes you have made over the past 3 weeks to help manage your symptoms and overall health moving forward.

Physical Activity

Type of Activity:

Duration:

Intensity:

☐ Low ☐ Moderate ☐ High

Sleep

Quality of Sleep:

☐ Excellent ☐ Poor
☐ Good ☐ Very Poor
☐ Fair

Hours Slept:

____

____

____

Support System:

Stress Management Techniques:

Water Intake Tracker:

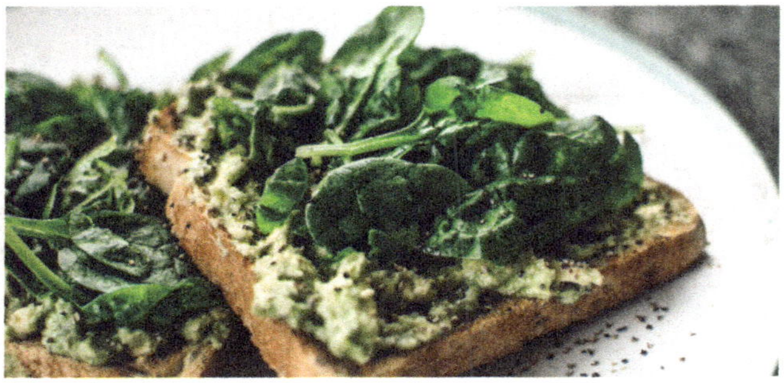

Overall Observations for the Day:

4 WEEK

Moving Forward

Symptom Management: Reflect on the dietary changes you have made over the past 3 weeks to help manage your symptoms and overall health moving forward.

Breastfeeding / Pumping Information

TIME	FEEDING / PUMPING		SLEEP OR ACTIVITY	BABY TOILETING	
	DURATION (Feeding)	AMOUNT (Bottle/ Pump)		PEE	POOP

Feelings & Observations

4
WEEK

Evening Reflections

Declutter Your Mind

As the day ends, take a moment to ***reflect on your day,*** and use this space to ***declutter your mind.*** Jot down your thoughts, feelings, and any moments that stood out. ***Often referred to as a "brain dump,"*** it's a method to understand, process, and release lingering thoughts that have built up throughout the day. Doing so will help to reduce stress and pave the way for a more peaceful night.

Thoughts/feelings

Use this space to let go of everything on your mind and write down your thoughts and feelings (from fleeting thoughts to deepest emotions). Writing them down without feeling "judged" helps you understand your feelings and prevents nighttime overthinking as you drift off to sleep.

Highlights and Today's Wins

What made you smile, feel proud, or brought you a sense of accomplishment today? Celebrate even the smallest wins and what you are especially thankful for here.

Evening Reflections

4 WEEK

Declutter Your Mind

Steps to Prepare For Tomorrow

Consider today's challenges. Which moments or areas is there room for growth or change? What steps can you take for a "better" tomorrow?

Rate Your Day

How would you describe your day on a scale of 1 to 10?
Use the emojis below as a guide, with 1 representing a difficult day and 10 symbolising an exceptional one...

1	2	3	4	5	6	7	8	9	10

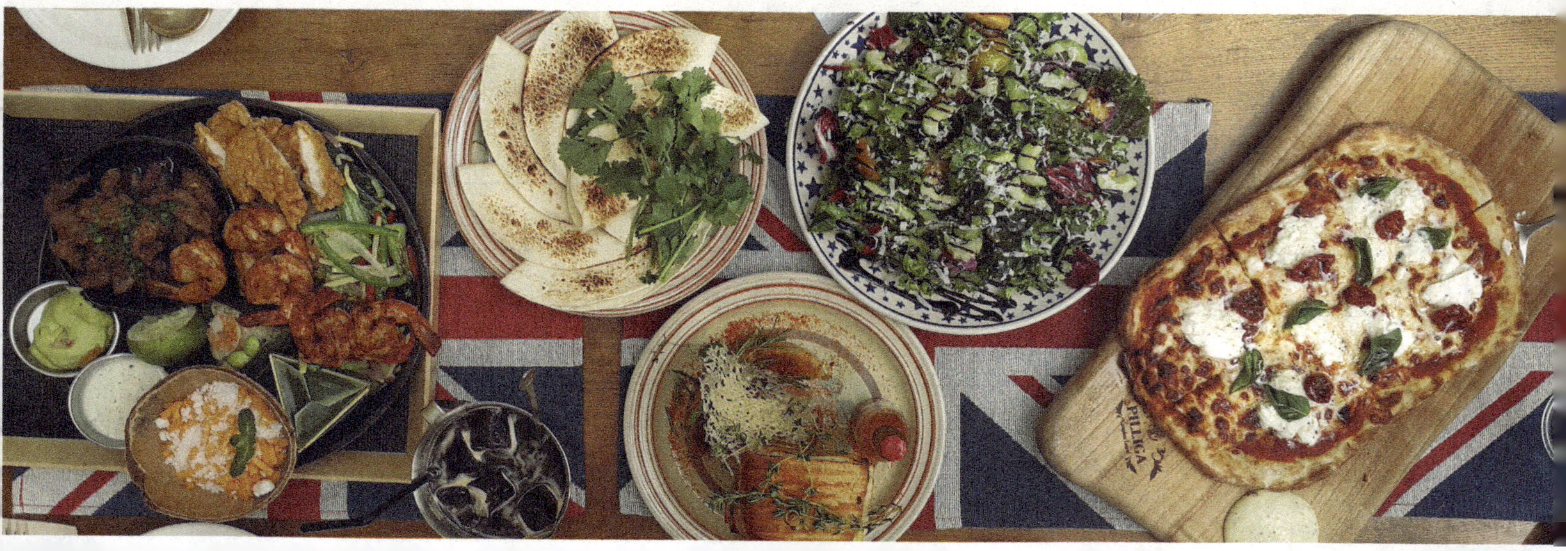

4 WEEK

Moving Forward

Symptom Management: Reflect on the dietary changes you have made over the past 3 weeks to help manage your symptoms and overall health moving forward.

Day 7

BREAKFAST

LUNCH

DINNER

SNACKS

DRINKS CONSUMED *(INCLUDING ALCOHOL)*

SUPPLEMENTS/MEDICATIONS TAKEN

HUNGER LEVELS BEFORE EATING

○ ○ ○ ○ ○ ○ ○ ○ ○ ○

1- NOT HUNGRY *10 - RAVENOUS*

MOOD BEFORE EATING

○ ○ ○ ○ ○

MOOD 1 HR AFTER EATING

○ ○ ○ ○ ○

MOOD 3 HRS AFTER EATING

○ ○ ○ ○ ○

BREAKFAST

LUNCH

DINNER

SNACKS

DRINKS CONSUMED *(INCLUDING ALCOHOL)*

SUPPLEMENTS/MEDICATIONS TAKEN

HUNGER LEVELS BEFORE EATING

○ ○ ○ ○ ○ ○ ○ ○ ○ ○

1- NOT HUNGRY *10 - RAVENOUS*

MOOD BEFORE EATING

○ ○ ○ ○ ○

MOOD 1 HR AFTER EATING

○ ○ ○ ○ ○

MOOD 3 HRS AFTER EATING

○ ○ ○ ○ ○

4 WEEK

Moving Forward

Day 7

Symptom Management: Reflect on the dietary changes you have made over the past 3 weeks to help manage your symptoms and overall health moving forward.

BREAKFAST

LUNCH

DINNER

SNACKS

DRINKS CONSUMED *(INCLUDING ALCOHOL)*

SUPPLEMENTS/MEDICATIONS TAKEN

HUNGER LEVELS BEFORE EATING

○ ○ ○ ○ ○ ○ ○ ○ ○ ○

1- NOT HUNGRY *10 - RAVENOUS*

MOOD BEFORE EATING

○ ○ ○ ○ ○

MOOD 1 HR AFTER EATING

○ ○ ○ ○ ○

MOOD 3 HRS AFTER EATING

○ ○ ○ ○ ○

BREAKFAST

LUNCH

DINNER

SNACKS

DRINKS CONSUMED *(INCLUDING ALCOHOL)*

SUPPLEMENTS/MEDICATIONS TAKEN

HUNGER LEVELS BEFORE EATING

○ ○ ○ ○ ○ ○ ○ ○ ○ ○

1- NOT HUNGRY *10 - RAVENOUS*

MOOD BEFORE EATING

○ ○ ○ ○ ○

MOOD 1 HR AFTER EATING

○ ○ ○ ○ ○

MOOD 3 HRS AFTER EATING

○ ○ ○ ○ ○

4
WEEK

Moving Forward

Symptom Management: Reflect on the dietary changes you have made over the past 3 weeks to help manage your symptoms and overall health moving forward.

Observations

- [ ] Bloating
- [ ] Energy Spike
- [ ] Irritability
- [ ] Headache
- [ ] Skin Reaction
- [ ] Nausea
- [ ] Vomiting
- [ ] Constipation
- [ ] Diarrhea
- [ ] Gas
- [ ] Other *(space for them to explain)*

Perimenopausal/Menopausal Symptoms

Symptoms Experienced

- [ ] Hot Flashes
- [ ] Sweating
- [ ] Night Sweats
- [ ] Anxiety
- [ ] Bloating
- [ ] Fatigue
- [ ] Gas
- [ ] Brain Fog
- [ ] Poor Concentration
- [ ] Mood Swings
- [ ] Cravings
- [ ] Sleep Disturbances
- [ ] Vaginal Dryness
- [ ] Headache
- [ ] Other (please explain)

- [ ] Mild
- [ ] Moderate
- [ ] Severe

Duration of Symptoms

- [ ] 5 Mins
- [ ] 15 Mins
- [ ] 1 Hour

New Symptoms:

Please explain

Observations:

Please explain

4 WEEK

Moving Forward

Symptom Management: Reflect on the dietary changes you have made over the past 3 weeks to help manage your symptoms and overall health moving forward.

Physical Activity

Type of Activity:

Duration:

Intensity:

☐ Low ☐ Moderate ☐ High

Sleep

Quality of Sleep:

☐ Excellent ☐ Poor
☐ Good ☐ Very Poor
☐ Fair

Hours Slept:

Support System:

Stress Management Techniques:

Water Intake Tracker:

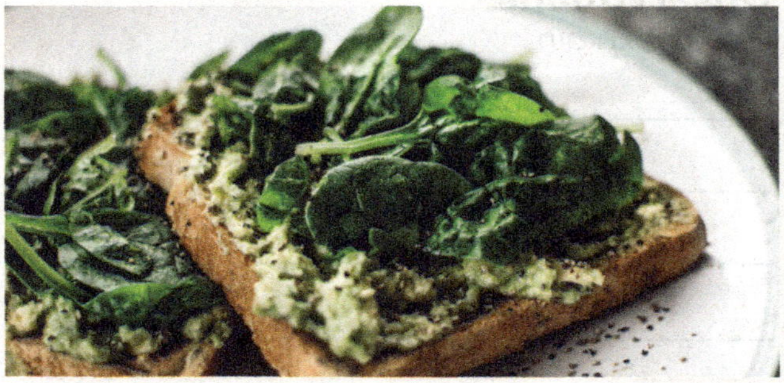

Overall Observations for the Day:

4 WEEK

Moving Forward

Symptom Management: Reflect on the dietary changes you have made over the past 3 weeks to help manage your symptoms and overall health moving forward.

Breastfeeding / Pumping Information

TIME	FEEDING / PUMPING		SLEEP OR ACTIVITY	BABY TOILETING	
	DURATION (Feeding)	AMOUNT (Bottle/ Pump)		PEE	POOP

Feelings & Observations

4
WEEK

Evening Reflections
Declutter Your Mind

As the day ends, take a moment to ***reflect on your day,*** and use this space to ***declutter your mind.*** Jot down your thoughts, feelings, and any moments that stood out. ***Often referred to as a "brain dump,"*** it's a method to understand, process, and release lingering thoughts that have built up throughout the day. Doing so will help to reduce stress and pave the way for a more peaceful night.

Thoughts/feelings

Use this space to let go of everything on your mind and write down your thoughts and feelings (from fleeting thoughts to deepest emotions). Writing them down without feeling "judged" helps you understand your feelings and prevents nighttime overthinking as you drift off to sleep.

____
____
____
____
____
____

Highlights and Today's Wins

What made you smile, feel proud, or brought you a sense of accomplishment today? Celebrate even the smallest wins and what you are especially thankful for here.

____
____
____
____
____
____
____

4 WEEK Evening Reflections
Declutter Your Mind

Steps to Prepare For Tomorrow

Consider today's challenges. Which moments or areas is there room for growth or change? What steps can you take for a "better" tomorrow?

Rate Your Day

How would you describe your day on a scale of 1 to 10?
Use the emojis below as a guide, with 1 representing a difficult day and 10 symbolising an exceptional one...

1	2	3	4	5	6	7	8	9	10

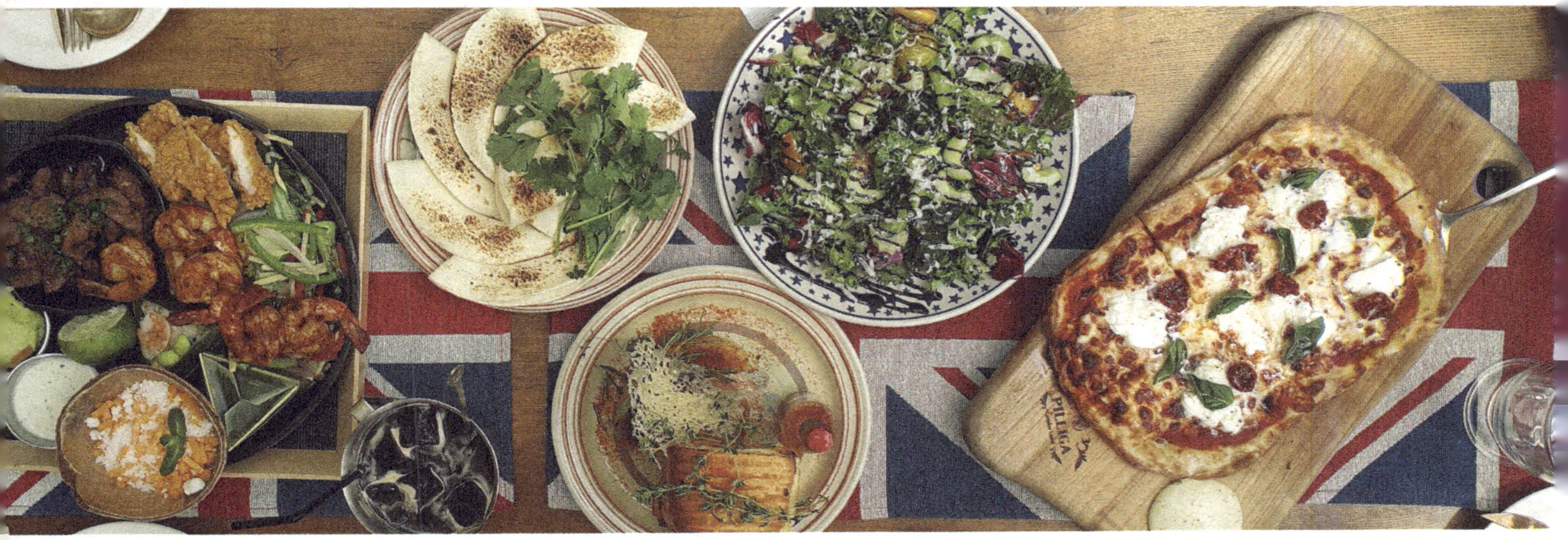

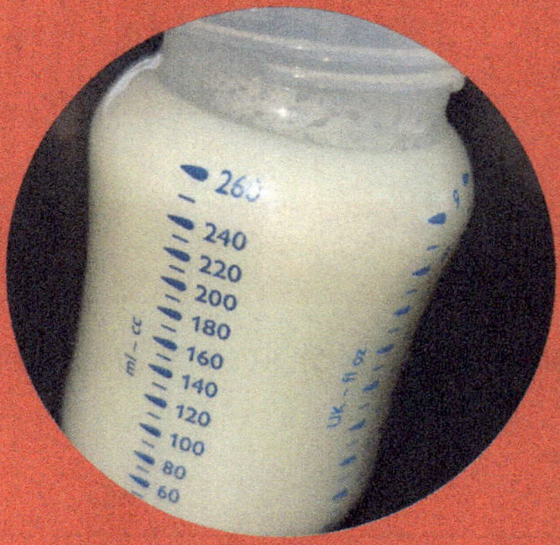

TAHLIA'S RESULTS JUST 3 WEEKS AFTER WORKING WITH KELLY WITHIN THE MAKE MORE MILK METHOD PROGRAM

"

The Make More Milk Method saved my breastfeeding journey!
I was struggling with under supply, I was exhausted and was so worried my baby girl was starving. I thought I had tried everything, until I found this program.

I was hesitant that the recipes wouldn't suit a family, but they were loved by the whole household.

My supply increased drastically!
I have been able to feed my daughter for 5 months so far and have enough milk in the freezer for at least 2 months worth of feeds, which is something I could never have imagined being able to do after the rocky start we had to breastfeeding!!

SCAN TO LEARN MORE ABOUT THE MAKE MORE MILK METHOD

SCAN ME

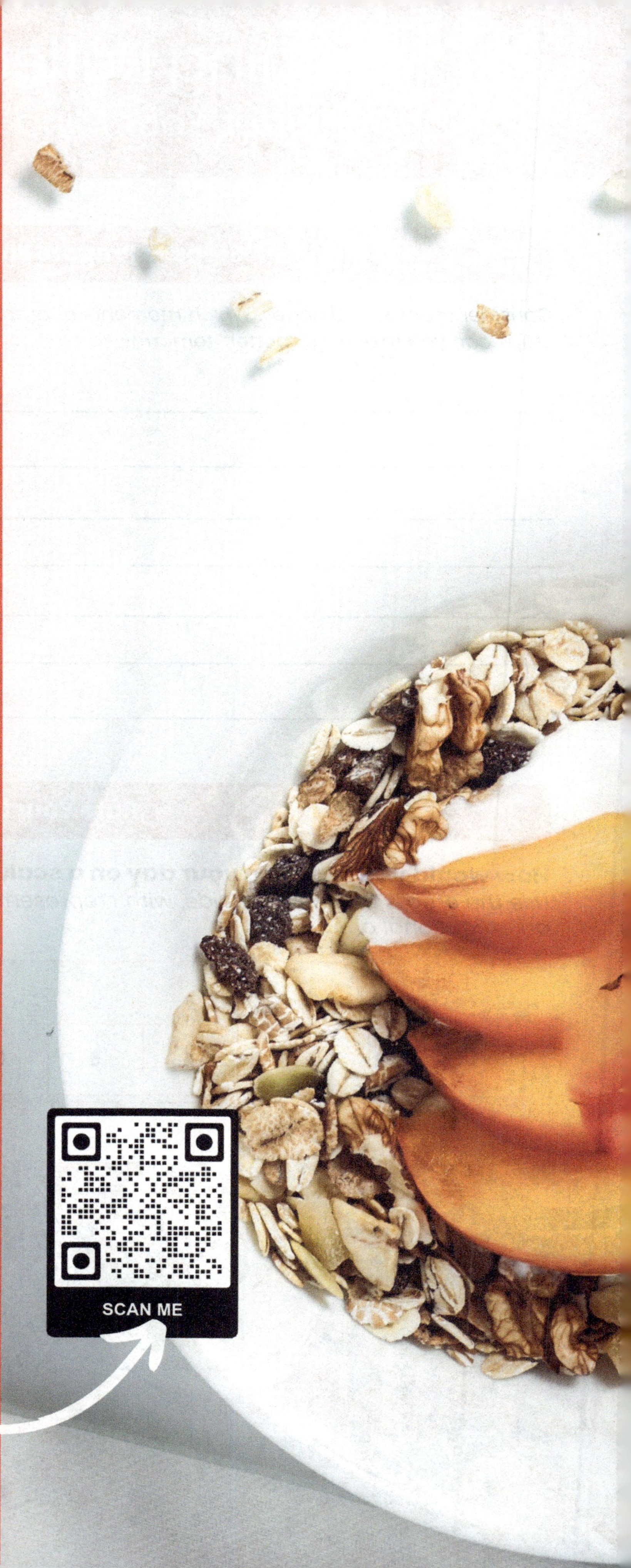

Made in the USA
Monee, IL
02 November 2026

67385956R00116